1

Finn Thoresen

Does the riddle of cancer have a solution?

Introduction to an exceptional treatment

Finn Thoresen

Does the riddle of cancer have a solution?

Introduction to an exceptional treatment

Second edition

Idéa cover: Finn Thoresen
Cover: Designlaboratoriet
Cover photo: Erling Halvorsen
The book is printed with Times New Roman

Translation from Norwegian to English

Eve Maria Thoresen

© 2016 Stiftelsen Robin H. org. nr. 977151937
ISBN-13: 978-1533190000 (CreateSpace-Assigned)

Published in cooperation with TheMa Forlag

Contents

Part IV
Status quo or a peaceful revolution?

Appendix

Postscript

Notes

Introduction to the first edition

To you who have the power to change

This English version of the book is a translation of a non-commercial first edition. In this second edition, a postscript written by the researcher, Are Thoresen, is added.

The intention of the publication was at first to inform leading politicians and other decision makers in the health field of new knowledge about prevention and life-saving treatment developed in Norway.

My contact with Health Department and The Office of the Prime Minister has given positive results which hopefully can be described in a third edition when our struggle for having Are Thoresens method or methods (a new or improved method for curing cancer is under development and presented in the postscript) will be tested in Norwegian hospital(s).

It seemed to be the correct first step that the information became known to people on the level where fundamental reforms to the general population are adopted.

The prevention effect of D-vitamin is also world-wide known, but it is few people who is aware of how much it would prevent the population from having a cancer diagnosis.

If this knowledge of how to prevent and how to cure cancer leads to practice, it will in addition to saving many lives and much suffering also provide significant savings to the health budget. Improvements may include preventive measures to minimize cost to the public and effective curative treatment that normally will not require hospitalization, but can be performed by general practitioners and oncologists with the necessary additional training. The method is also effective against advanced cancer with metastasis, and has saved the lives of a significant number of terminal (dying or doomed) patients.

7

Norwegian scientific research at the highest international level means that Norway can become a leader who leads the way to reversing the epidemic development of cancer diseases and reduce mortality significantly.

What has so far prevented this new knowledge to be implemented into practice, have been formulated by one of Norway's most internationally renowned cancer researchers[1], Johan Moan, in a conversation with the book's author. Moan is a professor in physics at the University of Oslo and head of the department of radiation biology at the Norwegian Radium Hospital. With his group of researchers[2], he is a key participant in one of the largest international networks in non-commercial cancer research. Moan asks one of the most important questions this book tries to answer: " Why am I, after a long research career with consistent recognition for my contributions, opposed by those who administer *consensus* within the health care system, just because I wanted to educate the Norwegian research community on important research findings not previously known? Why should this be kept secret and not disclosed to the medical profession[3], when this is vital information for the part of the medical community that would have put the knowledge into practice in the prevention and treatment?

Moan explains his use of the term consensus as *the majority of those who manages partly out-dated Cancer Research and deny the truths that have recently been published by a number of studies of the highest quality.*

Similar resistance was also experienced by a yet unknown researcher, Are Thoresen, but over a much longer period of time. Already thirty years ago, he discovered an effective, non-patentable and health-promoting treatment method that has helped some 700 Norwegian cancer patients, people and animals, and an unknown number in many other countries. There is today sixty clinics using this method with exceptional good results.

The method is based on the medical knowledge that *our immune system is multifaceted, and consists of different autonomic parts[4]* - a ground-breaking discovery at the time and which has recently become a recognized medical knowledge. The treatment strengthens that part of the immune system that inhibits or stops cancer development in healthy people. In most cases it can induce an immediate reversal of the disease.

While Thoresen is thwarted in Norway, his research and clinical outcomes are highly valued in the "world at large". Here I will mention two specific examples:

> • Two years after Thoresen was teaching a group of Canadian doctors about the method, it was presented in a *peer-reviewed[5]* journal.
> • Three years later, in the spring 2012, he was awarded a medal for his efforts to cure cancer in animals at the Veterinary University of Vienna. He was the annual congress' main lecturer.

While the method has gradually become widespread on five continents and his own book that describes it, is available in six languages, this year in Norway several attempts have been made to stop a study on dogs organized by Telemark University College, despite the fact that it meets the requirements for scientific evidence of the method's effectiveness. The unusual circumstances surrounding the preparation for the experiment is described in the book's epilogue.

In my view, the method should be subjected to scientific testing on humans, and the book shows how this can be done in several ways without coming into conflict with the ethical requirements to implement the authorized treatment[6]. The method can also be tested on terminal patients who are no longer offered hospital treatment, to verify the clinical results reported from many countries and from Thoresen´s own clinic about the effect on this population. Some examples from colleagues abroad are referenced in the book and in the appendix.

This can be done now - *if Parliament decides that the allegations the book presents should be tested by scientific control, so that the results can be published in a peer review journal.*

It is this book's assertion that if Moan and Thoresen´s knowledge[7] is applied, this will reduce the need for cancer researchers, oncologists, hospital-beds, costly medications and supplies - everything that has made cancer care into one of the states budget´s largest expenditure. That is; if the effect of Thoresens method does not change.
To everybodys great surprice this happened in the early part of 2014. This is described in the new chapter "Postscript" .

oOo

If there is not enough time to read the whole book, I suggest reading the chapters which, either in their entirety or selected parts, were conveyed by Sonja Mandt (Labor Party represent in the Parliament) before the election in the autumn 2013 to health politically engaged members of parliament on both sides in political opinions. Naturally enough, these selected chapters have a special academic policy significance and consists of a more concentrated introduction to what this is about. These are:

> **Chapter 2**, "The author's voice", is a short, focused supplement to this introduction - focused on the book's background and intention, while the next:

> **Chapter 3**,"The riddle and the solution", goes straight into the basic theme: Why have we not long ago found cancer disease´s "penicillin" - and where/how to look for it?

> **Chapter 10**, "Back to the patient diary. An epitome", in Part III is a concentrate of own experiences with the treatment, described in parallel (sequential) with the laboratory research based on Thoresen´s treatment method.

Chapter 12, "Anecdotal healings and natural cancer treatment", describes important discoveries that prevent and cure cancer.

Chapter 14, "Statistics as a witness of truth", refers key facts about the evolution of the disease, research and treatment.
Chapter 16,"An evaluation of Thoresen´s research" describes in more detail the new, effective curative treatment.
Chapter 25, "A highly unexpected change in the effect of the Method" describes in detail the totally unexpected change in the curative effect of the treatment in 2014.

On behalf of the Foundation Robin H[8]
and TheMa Forlag

Playa Del Cura, Spain, 11th of March 2016

Finn Thoresen

Part I

The riddle and the solution

1. A new beginning. From the first pages of a cancer patient's diary

Here, there
and
everywhere

Lennon/McCartney

It had been a long day. It began at the interface between winter and spring, and became the first early summer afternoon in my new life. I am at home at my own place, the main character both in my new life and in this story. A glance at the calendar shows the fourteenth of April two thousand and seven.

oOo

The morning stroll to the mailbox was lit by both sun and snow patches, and the meeting between the morning, the skin and the other senses piqued the annual uncertainty whether this really was a late winter day or a long- awaited spring day. It would remain to be seen.

This day was not like any other day, and I had a heightened awareness of what was closest to me – my mere existence, the weather and the sensations I met the world with in the opening of a new day.

Today the world was a little bit closer than usual, and I was absolutely sure I belong here.

For me it became the opposite for what is further away, where there is a distance or intermediaries/a mediator. What was not quite close, it was quite distant today, and I had little enjoyment of local news. I forgot all the time what I had just read, I had to read it again - because I failed to displace the notion that I would soon be getting a cold metal tool inserted deep into the body.

I set down my newspaper and remained seated as I envied those who could continue to be deeply involved in the question of whether this was the day when winter ended or spring began, and who could share the joy of the morning and keep focus on what dedicated representatives of the city's politicians, police, business community and cultural workers - and others who shared their views on this and that with the other subscribers of the daily newspaper.

What was stuck in my head was that I in scant three hours would get advanced technology through the hole in the body that I have so far had the least interest to explore. I've never seen it or cared about it, until it eventually forced me to take it seriously.

For nearly two years there have been signs of deviation of varying inconvenience around and within this opening. In depressed moments it had given me serious concerns.

In the beginning, like most would, I thought that this was transient. It was not. It was worsening - and confusing. Alternately threatening, fatal, alternately with a fuzzy prognosis and something that not really belonged to the present, but a hypothetical future.

The transient, serious concerns became less transient and more serious, which meant that one day I took the courage and told my dear E. that I over time had registered disturbing changes in my digestion.

When I had told the whole story, I knew that there was no turning back. This was definitely not going to go away by itself, and I did as I was told: make an appointment with my GP and got it sometime in early summer 2006.

oOo

The first time I was at the hospital, in the late 50s, it was called Tønsberg Hospital. When I a few years ago, visited the hospital on my own behalf, it had increased to at least twice the size and renamed Vestfold Central Hospital. Now it has at least doubled again and is called SIV, short for Vestfold Hospital, which may indicate that it will soon become the only hospital in the county. Although it has

16

grown into an entirely different order than it was fifty years ago, on the basis of the need for hospital treatment it has diminished. Growing up, I never heard of waiting lists for treatment or corridor patients. I realized after signing up with my GP that the necessary assistance needed when you are ill has become a limited resource when after a surprisingly long wait I received a call from the hospital telling me that I had a legal right to treatment after three months, but they could not provide it. There was not enough capacity in the hospital to ensure me my legal rights to hospital treatment. When asked how long I had to wait, I was told that it was impossible to say. The caller said I could choose if I would wait until there was space in Tønsberg, or that I could contact other hospitals to check if it was availability elsewhere in the country.

I was not in the mood to call around to hospitals in other parts of the country.

For fifteen years I had pushed my body to and above the borderline with work. It was natural enough that my head let me know this, and it was also in the head that it first became apparent, and where the noticeable changes occurred: confusion, irritation, pain and a recurring need to slow the pace down to almost no speed at all. After ten years of balancing on this line and repeatedly falling on the wrong side, and where I almost daily had to oppose the head's inclination to want to lie down on a pillow instead of continuing to give impetus to new actions, I was sent by my doctor to Granli, one branch of what was not yet SIV but still Vestfold Central Hospital and who had as specialty to assess possible Alzheimer's and similar issues.

I did not have Alzheimer's or similar issues. On the contrary, I was considered to be psychological, neurological and intellectual okay. But something - which at that time was a little unclear what it could be - had for a long time *gone hot* and become so *burned out* (contemporary speech in the absence of a medical term) which, according to the doctor one was able to be before one was no longer able to resist its head's inclination, perhaps even having to turn off the lights to escape the feeling of passing out.

The doctor pointed to the relatively modest knowledge about this condition and predicted that I had between one and ten years to recapture almost normal mental and intellectual capacity - if I stopped doing everything that had brought me into the outer limits of meaningful existence.

Between one and ten years, I thought, and went home without any special plan to stop some of what I had vague suspicions could have led to this point. This existence often stood as a steep wall without windows and doors in front of me. What could cause it to flatten out after I moved into it, as I was used to it doing automatically the first half of my life, *what I'm up to now had considered about half*, I had no clear thoughts about.

It later was described as *chronic fatigue syndrome* or *ME* (short for *myalgic encephalomyelitis*), followed me faithfully like a dog the next few years. There was never any lasting improvement, probably because I had so meaningful and, based on self-assessment, responsible tasks that I did not steer clear from even though I was convinced that these could be a partial cause of the health problems. Every time I was noticeably less afflicted, I thought that now I was back in normal shape again, and was soon seated in front of the PC 15 minutes too long, made the problematic phone-call or went to the meeting that sent me back to strict rationing of the mental powers.

There was a big difference between the seasons. In the late summer/early fall, the time where I got the phone call from the hospital, I was up to 90 % able-bodied - assuming I did not read a single book, wrote articles for my own sake, made phone-calls I did not absolutely have to make, and so on. The three or four least sunny months of the year I was down to between ten present and zero of my normal work capacity, and I cheated my way through the daily tasks, partly by getting mail and other paper work done in the evening after a half bottle of wine, partly by pushing all work that could be pushed towards the spring thaw, and partly by sneaking south toward living nature and life-giving sun but since it was too little with the few weeks I could get E. with me, I created tasks that demanded that I travelled southward to solve them.

I wanted to feel as well as possible when I eventually got the message that I was ill, and so far the timing had been good and by this I mean seriously ill, not just burnt out or other unpleasantness that is not worth putting down in writing.

After the phone-call from the hospital - where they regretted that they could not give me the examination I had a legal claim to - I realized that I approached the time when it would no longer be good timing, when I no longer had the inner strength I thought I would need when I very probably would have to start the strength-consuming work having cancer means for most people. Going into the darkness of autumn with increasing fatigue and in battle with health bureaucracy to expedite a possible devastating diagnosis both my intuition and my common sense made such strong objection to that I let it be.

I went instead to a medical practitioner, originally veterinarian, who treats humans and animals and has a background in both school-medical and so-called alternative therapies. His specialty is acupuncture. Are Thoresen is his name, Are Simeon Thoresen, who had earlier saved me from both debilitating back problems and something I many years ago had perceived as an acute, serious health problem. If it really was serious, I'll never know because the recovery began after only one acupuncture-treatment.

This was not something I could address on the phone, so I went to his small clinic in Sandefjord, where a few days a week he changed hat and replaced the veterinary practice with human medicine.

oOo

After many years with an amateur interest of health issues, where the disease complex of *cancer* oddly enough was the area I had been most involved in, I found that the diagnosis was one of the most dangerous aspects of the disease. What preoccupied me was the emotional and psychological reactions the notions related to the diagnosis and symptoms triggered in the patients, and that I had considered as potentially as dangerous for further growth in tumours and spread to other parts of the organism as other known factors. Instead of being a warning about the need for change, as I believe most disease symptoms should be understood as, the diagnosis is for many a notice of premature death. Getting confirmation of these symptoms, I thought could be a huge additional problem that in many cases may weaken the ill person 's own ability to help themselves through the disease in a targeted and meaningful way. I had come to the conclusion that if I received the worst case scenario diagnosis, while I was already feeling down and further weakened by my depression tendencies of the past two or three years in addition to the ME symptoms, I would really be almost finished before I even got started on any new treatment.

Not exactly a desirable situation, and in my imagination I had long envisioned a period of dressing gown and slippers, where I toddled around - barely on my feet after an emaciating and further draining medical treatment. Maybe a short time with a clean bill of health and a supposed recovery before it popped up again - here, there and everywhere.

Here, there and everywhere by Beatles became a kind of comfortless comfort in my head every time I pictured the future´s most challenging scenario: *No future whatsoever*.

I let the hustle and bustle of E. pass through one ear and out of the other, until it began to dawn again, both inside and out, in the beginning of March the following year. I called the hospital again and asked if they had forgotten about me. Possibly they had, because suddenly there was available capacity, or it had just become my turn, and only two days later I received a letter in the mail that I had an appointment at the Department of Gastroenterology for colonoscopy with Chief Physician *Arne Drivenes*.

oOo

Vestfold Hospital is bright, open and welcoming. It has a good atmosphere, although the weight and uncertainty that characterises some of the patients meeting you in the foyer, can easily lead to a depression in the mood. Despite meeting with bandaged and wheelchair seated patients already outside the entrance, patients who apparently had no better place to smoke, and in spite of the seriousness of my own errand, I preserved my close to nature ambience I had with me from the possible spring day or the very last day of winter in South-East of Norway. The innate, distance-creating ability people have, meant that I saw myself from the outside, just as if I had been there in the more privileged position as a visitor.

Displacement psychologists call it, but it is at least a natural process, far from an artificial displacement as you get from valium and the like.

When I passed the foyer and followed the arrow to the Department of Gastroenterology towards the stairs to the first floor, I reflected on the positive impression I had of the hospital, if it was something which was already imprinted in the walls, a phrase which in this case refers to a hospital culture with great ability for care-taking, or whether this impression mostly had to do with myself - if I during the winter had managed to process the notion of myself in a dressing gown and toddling emaciated off to the newspaper kiosk ...

I will no longer drag it out or get side-tracked:

Immediately after the instrument was inserted and the screen was turned on to the left of me, which both gastroenterology specialist Arne Drivenes and I stared at, I noticed a lump of irregular "meat" which I immediately realised was foreign to this area of myself. I looked to the right, at Drivenes, who probably did not received the same extra heartbeat as I did, but looked just as worried, and by his expression and bringing the instrument back and forth in this area confirmed that this was a large - at least it was very big on the screen - unattractive and totally superfluous collection of formless and aimless cell tissue.

oOo

While I waited for an appointment at the hospital, I had chosen to seek out Thoresen to see if there was some truth in what I heard from one of his patients: that he had developed a treatment that was beneficial for cancer patients.

It turned out to be not only correct, but that he had for almost twenty-five years practiced the method on both humans and animals. It was surprising that this was not more known, not only because of the good results over such a long time, but also from what he told me about the treatment's prevalence in many countries and several continents.

However, there was one crucial obstacle at that time preventing him from giving me this treatment.

> - Before you receive a medical diagnosis, all I can do is to treat the nervousness in the lower part of the colon.
> - *Why not?*
> - If you have cancer, it is important to know in which organ or in which part of the organism it originated from. A large tumour may be an overgrown child of a smaller tumour that first occurred elsewhere, but has not led to noticeable problems. There are different methods to stimulate the body's own ability to self heal depending on where the disease started. The immune system is multifaceted and the different parts are autonomic as you know.
> - *And the cause or the deficit need not be at the same place as where we notice the symptoms?*
> - Right. But you will still notice an improvement in the bowel function during the first few months, which in any event would be beneficial, even if it turns out you have colon cancer.

Thoresen had neither seemed surprised or particularly worried about my message, which I attributed to his professionalism more than a lack of empathy for his patient's health problem. Either way I understood it as he was not able to ascertain whether I had cancer or

22

not, but "only" discover if there was something wrong with my energetic cycle. What he eventually found, he said nothing about. Although Thoresen had previously told me a little about the mechanisms of acupuncture, my general knowledge in this field was so bad that I could not get a clear understanding of what he communicated to me through the observations he made using what acupuncturists describe as *pulse diagnosis*[12]. One main reason is probably that the acupuncture treatment´s effects are originating from an "*area*" - a non-physical element - in our organism, that our own medical science does not even accept the existence of. Human and warm-blooded animal´s energetic cycle, which Indians and especially the Chinese have based their medical research upon through at least five millennia, has never been any ingredient in our general knowledge. Therefore, it is difficult to accept that this may have a different impact on disease other than in the form of *placebo*, which is the technical term. It is this energetic cycle, not the cardiovascular system, that the acupuncturist who masters this diagnostic method, "take the pulse" of.

Thoresen gave me a treatment aimed at curbing the turmoil in the digestive system and suggested that it could take as much as two months before a noticeable improvement would occur. He wished me good luck with the colonoscopy and said he could give a more specific treatment when I had ascertained what was physically wrong with the digestion system.

Two days later - not two months, as Thoresen had suggested - there was a noticeable change. The morning ritual was far more relaxed. Although the day still began with a trip or two to the WC, I could for the first time in over six months have breakfast coherent, and quickly was able to half my toilet visits.

Whether it was the acupuncture needle that had taken the edge off the morning unrest, or I was better because I imagined that the treatment would work (placebo) or something else, other symptoms also became so much better during the autumn and winter, that, which I previously judged to be of pencil thickness, when I occasionally took courage and turned around to check, now was more of a fountain pen, the slightly chubby, expensive variety, which now barely exists, but some of us who have seen better days was fortunate enough to get as a Christmas gift even before we left primary school.

oOo

A few months later I decided that Thoresen had already taken my concerns more seriously than he expressed back in the autumn of 2006. For when in the spring of 2007 I found it necessary to visit him again in connection with the health, I had a few follow-up questions and he told me what name the ancient Chinese had set at the point where he had placed the needle.

> - *This is a so-called universal point, which in some places is also referred to as a survival point.*

2. The author's voice

Three years after I was given a serious cancer diagnosis, I began to write a book. It became a very different book than the patient diary I wrote to document the extraordinary course of the disease. A more *subject-influenced* book - I have to describe it in this way, as I do not have any formal medical training. There has also been a goal to reach as many people as possible that are affected by cancer: equally to those affected by the disease as healthcare professionals and researchers who attempt to cure or alleviate it.

Ideally I would like, however, to start a dialogue with those who makes decisions in Norwegian health policy, so that the problematic conditions within cancer care this book reveals, can be followed up and changed through appropriate measures. The ambition to reach within this broad catchment area has naturally enough led to some compromises, mostly so obvious that here I just want to mention that for me it has been the most problematic: The hardest thing has been to include me and my story instead of anonymising "the patient" and it has for a long time been hard to do. I have never had any desire to extradite myself and my life, and least of all in terms of a patient 's history.

I have read some books by so-called *alternative* therapists/authors, but rarely seen the purpose of the patient stories that almost always belong in these books and in different ways stand in opposition to *authorised medicine*[13]. However, there is a crucial difference between the present patient history and those I have read. My patient diary is actually built on a skeleton of medical records from the hospitals I visited and medical records from my GP – as I collectively describes as the *case journal*.

The latter is full of documentation from physicians, oncologists, surgeons, radiologists, pathologists, a cancer researcher, a practitioner in social medicine and most importantly: the results conveyed by all the technology in an optimal objective and scientific way confirms that what I write about my illness is true. The reflections concerning this are of course subjective, but - based on irrefutable facts. These constitute what I call the patient diary and which is referred from and is given a summary of later in this book.

My patient history does not describe something alternative, but rather something *novel*: a new form of healing cancer based on a combination of millennia-old medical science and new scientific knowledge and technology. As shown by both the patient diary and the present book this is not a formal collaboration - yet - neither a collaboration between representatives of the two different medical sciences. I forced cooperation upon the authorised health care system, indirectly and through the independent choices I took after I was diagnosed.

What I see as most important by a formalised cooperation is that it is an absolute necessity for both the involved medical sciences if our fellow citizens should be offered the same opportunities for treatment that not only I, but hundreds[14] of cancer patients worldwide have now been able to experience.

This collaboration is described here in general and in principle both as a possible target for a comprehensive national cancer care and a possible model for other countries' cancer care. As indicated above the cooperation with the hospitals involved got a "difficult birth" and is far from exemplary - with the exception of the technology delivered which is neutral. I saw therefore the need for a textbook that goes far beyond this single process, and is the reason I let the patient diary be and started the present book. It does not deny its origin, but is only modestly based on my specific experiences, my quotes from the patient diary and my medical history. If the general and fundamental questions this book addresses arouse the attention that I think this ground-breaking, Norwegian method of treatment for cancer deserves, I will continue where I left off in the first chapter and tell the whole story of my illness and healing as I and the involved physicians have observed it.

Details of what makes a partnership between east and west, old and new, authorised and "alternative" medical knowledge to an absolute necessity to allow the new treatment method to be used in a responsible manner, is described in chapter 6 ("The bridges").

The most important thing with the new treatment method is that it is mainly oriented towards *healing*, and if this fails, to raise the *quality of life* as a cancer patient. As known, all authorised medical treatments used today - surgery, chemotherapy and radioactive irradiation – cause temporary or permanent poorer quality of life. What is not as well known, is that these methods simply leads to *an extension of life* and rarely to a permanent healing. This was also completely unknown to me until I thoroughly investigated the cancer statistics for the last fifty years[15], which was necessary to fulfil the ambition to provide a broad documented description of both the history and status of the forms of treatment which have an impact on the choices of cancer patients ultimately does for themselves.

    The issue of patients' own choices are virtually non-existent and a non-issue in cancer treatment. All important decisions are made centrally from the Norwegian Radium Hospital. This is in itself no medical sensation, but that patients only slightly or not at all are consulted, was an unexpected experience for me. I came to the conclusion that this must be something special concerning cancer, possibly rooted in ancient traditions, that make it so that patients are seldom aware that it is they themselves who actually have the right to make the final choice of treatment in some extent the form of treatment, and that choice should *not* be taken for them. At least as long as they are "sane" as my oncologist with an undercurrent of humour described me as in a letter to the Norwegian Radium Hospital - probably as a reminder that as long as we are able to make choices and not under guardianship, it is we ourselves who choose.

Because cancer statistics show that what has been achieved mainly is an extension of life, with some important exceptions for some less common cancers, it is all the more evident that the cancer riddle, the core of the problem complex, must be disclosed to liquidate the cancer wildfire in the civilised world.

    Hence the title of the book and of the next chapter.

3. The riddle and the solution

What is the most remarkable, and simultaneously being the solution to the problem is the following: In most science it is recognised that all our inventions like night vision, sonar, airplanes, x-ray and more are already invented by nature. We just need to emulate it. If one in energy production would mimic photosynthesis, one would also have solved the problem here. In medicine, we know how everything works correctly (physiology). Likewise, we know how things go wrong (pathology), and attempting to find methods to correct what went wrong (therapy). What is missing is that we do not recognise, or research how the body itself has already constructed ingenious mechanisms at several levels to correct what has gone wrong. Medical research has rarely utilised that the body itself has already engineered medicines for all diseases.

Thoresen's written response after reading "The riddle and the solution"

Western medicine has over the last few centuries cracked the codes for the most serious and life-threatening diseases - at least in terms of the symptoms. The cancer riddle, however, remained a mystery, despite the enormous technical and financial resources that are spent on cancer research throughout the history of modern medicine.

Not everyone is aware that from the very embryonic stage mutations[16] occur in the organism that will lead to the formation of cancerous tumours unless something stops and clears away these incipient faulty structures. This work is carried out continuously by something in our body, and when that something at some point stops

29

working for more and more of us, this can lead to life-threatening cancer.

To find and understand what the body itself performs, or which substance(s) produced by your body that continually stop mutations, will be a first and crucial step toward a final solution. If you succeed in either copying these processes or helping the body to restore them, and you can repeat this on a large percentage of people with cancer, the cancer riddle will be solved.

oOo

After discussing this main question with an oncologist, Wenche Gustafson at Vestfold Hospital, and to the best of my ability to understand the key elements of modern cancer treatment and cancer research, I became aware that science has had, and still has, an exclusive focus on only one of the two main elements that the concept of the cancer puzzle can be divided into, namely

how things work correctly, and what have gone wrong.

Cancer research has a long tradition with attention to what has gone wrong. The research resources have consistently been directed solely against the symptoms[17]. This is usually about the last stage of cancer development, i.e. when it has gone wrong for so long that the tumour has become a threat to the surrounding tissues and organs, and ultimately for human life. It is not surprising that clinicians have shown the greatest interest in this aspect of the cancer problem, as they continuously acted to save as many lives as possible. But for an amateur it may seem strange that no research is increasingly focused on how things work correctly, in order just to help out or copy these parts of the processes.

Cancer research has over time acquired a lot of knowledge about what's going wrong and how it goes wrong, in order to develop methods to prevent it going wrong. It has proved to be very numerous and complex processes where errors can occur, and can be said to be partial causes of cancer. The question is whether this focus will ever succeed in reversing or stopping enough of these processes that it can turn people's rapidly increasing propensity to develop serious cancer.

One of the examples of how far research has come from this angle of attack, is a Danish research group that for years has worked from the realisation that what can go wrong, is very diverse, indeed, that the causes of disease can demonstrate individual differences. Therefore, their vision of the future is to create a medicine that is tailored to the individual patient, i.e. a medicine that targets the place where it has gone wrong, and specifically where these specific cell structures require repair.

For an amateur, this may seem like an endless task, and an obvious question is whether it will prove possible to make such a vision of the future into reality. Which leads to a new question: What will it cost to develop such a drug? Will anyone other than the world's wealthiest afford to buy it?

If the Danes are right, then what has gone wrong has proved to be so strongly associated with external causes and the individuals life cycle that ideally we need a specifically tailored medicine for every cancer patient to stop the process going wrong in a safe and effective way.

What is working correctly, however, is not controlled by the environment and individual development. It is part of man's innate luggage and is common to all. Whoever finds something which by nature itself stifle the disease in the bud or stimulate a body that has lost the ability to regain it, has found the medication for everyone.

oOo

If we move the focus from what has gone wrong to what is working correctly, we discover soon that a hundred years of neglect have left large white areas on the map of our ignorance, we did not even know was there. If we look to another science, geography, we are in a situation that is comparable to the time when the interior of Africa was just a huge, white and un-described area. Medically, we have barely become aware that Africa exists, in other words it means that the body´s self-healing is by far the most effective and simplest form

31

of cure for disease, and that it is possible to stimulate this healing method consciously and purposefully, both against specific disease states and prevention by effectively inhibit diseases from occurring. Eastern medicine in general has for many thousands of years explored self-healing and knew "Africa" like the back of their hand, figuratively speaking, at a time when Europeans had not even begun geographical exploration.

Thanks to biological and general medical research European medicine knows today much about natural, organic processes and how they are controlled. However, we are almost completely unaware of how organic processes can intervene where it has gone wrong, and restore the proper processes, and possibly repair the damage. But we know that it happens and we know that all modern medicine is completely at the mercy of such processes. How could we, for example perform surgery unless our organism on its own was able to heal the wounds surgeons inflict on the body during operations? We would bleed to death from the slightest abrasions if nothing were done from within the body itself to prevent it.

Why do we not know more of such processes, not even enough to be able to begin to develop methods or medications that help the organism to maintain these processes? Almost without exception, our methods and medicines puts an additional burden on organs like the liver, kidneys and heart, or they come in direct conflict with what is the center for natural healing processes - our own immune system.

There are at least two reasons for this lack of knowledge about what stops the dangerous mutations in our body, and thus is able to prevent the development of cancer in the majority of us. The first reason has to do with what is mentioned in the focus of the research. It has been devoted to tumours and combating them. The second reason springs directly out of the first one and is ethically motivated: it is in fact never been researched on other patients than those receiving the treatment that always has been considered the most effective and which consists of different forms of removal of symptoms - either by surgery, chemotherapy, radiation or various combinations of these

32

methods. For ethical reasons, it has not been possible to recommend patients to take the risk by retaining the symptoms through a research project. This has prevented scientists gaining knowledge about what happens in cancer cells and tumours in patients where the growth of tumours is either inhibited, halted, or where the tumours shrinks or even completely disappear through self- healing. Today there is only one medical term for the different forms of illness where cancerous tumours evolve significantly more favourable (for the patient) than can be expected from a medical, statistical background. All these cases have in common the term *anecdotal healing* - which in reality means that the healing has no known cause. What causes anecdotal healing, which in reality is a full recovery, medical science knows nothing about.

There are certainly patients who for various reasons have chosen not to implement the recommended cancer treatment, and one can imagine the possibility that some of these could be volunteers in a research context. To grapple with such research one must first overcome an active negativity within the authorised cancer treatment against the unauthorized (and illegal in Norway) treatment. On the one hand, such an attitude is necessary to prevent the spread of ineffective treatment of non-qualified therapists, but on the other hand, the same attitude prevent the spread of effective treatment by highly qualified clinicians and researchers.

For both effectively to prevent quacks and simultaneously encourage research in sectors where clinical results indicate that research can bear fruit requires an unprejudiced examination of what happens outside the authorised treatment procedures. Instead one has so far rejected all who do not follow the conventional medical research track. Subject to a possible exception in the form of a project under the University of Tromsø named NAFKAM (*National Research Center in Complementary and Alternative Medicine*). NAFKAM is the only institution of its kind in the western world of research and in June 2010 became an active partner with the UN agency WHO (World Health Organisation). If NAFKAM actually is completely open-minded in the study of other forms of research than the one based on a scientific perspective, has been controversial from the very inception, a discussion I do not have the qualifications to participate in.

In the next round these views raise the following question:

> *If someone through clinical practice can prove that he has found a method that stimulates the body's own way to stop the unwanted mutations, and can in many cases also demonstrate that he can reactivate this ability, where it is put out of action, will the Norwegian research community then be sufficiently open and unprejudiced so he gets the opportunity to show us in controlled trials - trials in which all the scientific world can keep an eye on - if he is really capable of this?*

4. Who is Are Thoresen?

Regarding Are Thoresen, I am full of respect. He is one of the most intriguing figures we have in Norwegian medical research today. And I find it very interesting that he, as a veterinarian, has raised the absolutely central question in medical science: Whether the doctor's intention is paramount to the effect of the medical treatment.

Vilhelm Schjelderup, doctor

First, a few words about the chapters in the book that describes the two scientists who set out to build a bridge between Eastern and Western world-views and these very different culture's medical traditions. My presentation of them evolved on its own term as I see them as very different "temperaments", as different as the scientific traditions they have chosen to bring their research tools from.

What the two have in common is that both have their schooling in the Western tradition, but has an individualistic and unconventional path from the school-bench and towards solving the tasks that the book talks about – as highly independent *scientists*.

Instead of promoting my own views or personal characteristics, I have chosen to introduce Thoresen as a professional. I will follow the preamble with another practitioner's review, and then I selected two texts where Thoresen provided a sketch of an academic self-portrait while approaching the core of medical beliefs of more universal character.

In part two I have referenced a conversation with Thoresen that connects his career to biography and personal characteristics, partly based on feedback I get from the reviews of others who know him, and partly from the conversation itself.

With Thoresen's research colleague, molecular biologist Sergio Manzetti, it was different. I think it was due to his immediate transparency, which invited to take part in and describe his personality in a more direct way. Because I had not met him and was therefore surprised, almost overwhelmed by the huge difference in expectations and preconceptions - from a mythical pre-review from those I had spoken to regarding his professional expertise, to the youthful fireworks that without superfluous introductions exposed himself and his strong views on medical research in our garden.

If anyone believes that I at certain points in the description of Sergio Manzetti in the book's third part I am exaggerating, then they are welcome to do so. Seen from my side it appeared impossible to use too strong a word to describe him, and with Thoresen it occurs some of the same difficulty - but with the opposite sign.

Thoresen is not only phlegmatic. He *is* the definition of phlegmatic: an impenetrable calm that I am not yet familiar with to such an extent that I can describe where it originates from. I have no doubt that he also has temperament. However, I restrict myself here to describe his professional side, where he rarely reviews the ups and downs with the fluctuating tone I had expected.

It is also what he has accomplished more than who he is, which is interesting to me. As I have not had contact with his professional opponents - which I suspect is opposed mainly because of lack of knowledge about his business – the representation is necessarily one-sided. His Irish colleague´s, Phil Rogers, review of him also says something about the difficulty associated with mapping Thoresen professional "universe", whose contents I can only express in a superficial and more widely accessible form.

Thoresen and Rogers are colleagues within the special branch of medicine termed as *veterinary acupuncture*. Thoresen has his basic medical studies from the Norwegian School of Veterinary Science, an education that is more similar to medical school than most people realise. Throughout his 60 years of life, he has schooled himself in what he has found interesting, perfecting so-called alternative therapies, where acupuncture in most cases, in light of the results he has achieved with his needles, has remained his preferred treatment of choice. Not primarily the method taught in educational institutions, but a development of this that has made him an internationally recognised researcher/lecturer in this special field.

One of the countless examples of his extensive travel throughout thirty years is that while this script is being prepared for release - we write today 7th of December 2013 – Thoresen is a guest lecturer at Murdoch University in Fremantle, Australia, by invitation of Professor Bruce Ferguson[18].

Because a lot of the innovations being made in the work with dogs and horses have direct transferability to the human organism, the human practice became not just a clinical utilisation, but a third field where his development of the acupuncture profession had beneficial effects in all directions. This is how his discovery of how to cure cancer in dogs and horses, also have benefitted a large number of people.

It must be emphasised that for Thoresen the animals are not merely laboratory animals with human health as the final goal. When it comes to other diseases, it may as well be dogs and horses that receive advantage of "attempts" tested on humans.

The following quote is a slightly shortened version of Rogers' review of Thoresen in the English translation of the latter's book in which he describes his medical thinking and methodology: *Veterinary Medicine: Complementary and Alternative Methods* (Amazon 2013).

> *"Holistic medicine as defined her by Are Thoresen, is especially occupied by four main factors in development of disease; (a) the predisposing factor, (b) the initiating factor, (c) the weak anatomical structure and (d) the syndrome.*
>
> * *The **predisposing factor (a)** is an inner unbalance, usually a **deficiency**, in one or more of the 12 main processes (meridians, organs).*

- *The **stressor** or **initiating factor (b)** is the external or internal **stress**, which trigger the already deficient internal process to collapse.*

In addition to these two main factors responsible for the development of disease, it will be important also to be able to consider

- *The **weak spot (c)**. This is the "Achilles-heel" of the organism, the **weak anatomical structure** or stressed part where any deficiency most probably will manifest itself.*
- *In this weak anatomical area the **syndrome (d)** will manifest. The syndrome is the material **manifestation of the disease**. The syndrome is not the disease itself, only the body's own manifestation of the inner deficiency. This manifestation is also very often the body's attempt to help the deficient inner process.*

The book discusses animals as sentient beings and criticises the adverse effects that human interaction inflicts on the health and welfare of their animals. It discusses acupuncture theory in detail, the 12 Channel-Organ Systems and their Processes, the Vessels, the Command Points and main Channel Points in humans, horses and dogs.

This is a subversive book. It recognises the strengths of ModMed but challenges its arrogance, its failure to address the basic causes of disease, its heavy reliance on therapies that merely suppress symptoms, and use of surgery when less invasive therapy could be successful. It recognises the innate superiority and wisdom of Holistic medicine but also its failures and weaknesses and its dependence on the ability of the body's adaptive systems to respond. No one system of medicine has, or is likely to have, all the answers to treat or prevent all disease. Although it does not say so explicitly, Holistic medicine implies that one can gain competence in medicine and healing only after long and broad study and experience, and that few people receive the gift of their mastery.

As thunder inevitably involves lightning (discharge of static electricity), Are's ideas will electrify readers whose minds are not insulated by the dull dead drapes of conventional medical thinking. He is the most amazing professional that I have had the privilege to know. He has been my friend and mentor for many years, but that was not always the case. I first heard him talk in 1986 at a European Veterinary Acupuncture Congress in Belgium. Then, I thought that he was crazy because his ideas of medicine and healing were so different from those of mainstream thought, and the success rates that he claimed were so much better than those that I could attain at that time. Later, I realised that my rejection of Are was a "mental knee-jerk" to the severe challenge that his ideas posed to my world-view. I swallowed my egotistical pride and asked if I could visit him to see his methods. Like St. Thomas, I was a doubter. I would not believe unless I could verify his claims for myself. Are agreed to one visit. That was the start of my un-blinding. Since then, I have stayed at his home many times and have talked to his animal-owners and his human patients. They confirmed that his methods are very successful in clinical practice.

In the spring of 2000, Are asked me if I would correct an English draft of this book. Not suspecting the amount of work involved, I agreed. I tore it apart line-by-line and emailed "my corrections", peppered with thousands of queries, to Are. He answered all of these and came to my home in late November to finalise the drafting. So I know this book like I know my hands! I have wrestled with it, mauled it, thrown it away and returned to it time and again. It still amazes me. It has assembled between two covers a wealth of knowledge that I have not seen anywhere before now. I believe that it will be seen as a key influence in the further development of holistic medicine.

Are has been my patient teacher for years; I have learned much from him. However, I suspect that his controversial ideas will scandalise many professionals who do not know him personally. Readers unfamiliar with acupuncture, holistic principles, or natural healing, will find his ideas very difficult initially. After a first reading of the book, if you are tempted to dismiss its ideas as crazy (my first reaction to meeting Are in 1986), I urge you to reconsider. Read it again! And if you do not understand it then, read and re-read it until you do. When you begin to realise and apply his wisdom in your practice, your life and your approach to healing will change; they will differ radically from what they were before.

As I grow older, I am increasingly aware of the meaning behind the myths of Plato's Cave, or the more modern version of the Three Blind Men and the Elephant. Those myths boil down to a debate about subjective versus objective truth. The grace and beauty of science could and should be the study of the natural world in the search for objective truth, and the practical application of that knowledge for the good of all.

Overall, the book inspires wonder and awe, which are the spice of life and the basis of spirituality. It is not "scientific" in the strict sense; indeed it has some ideas that I would reject on my knowledge of science. I must reserve judgement on those few areas but I am content to accept that Are's clinical experiences, described so well in this book, are true. Indeed, for several years I have used his thinking process and some of his acupuncture methods, with better results than I had attained beforehand. I wish Are, his loved ones and this book great success. May its controversial and profound ideas help you (the reader) and others as much as they have helped me."

Phil Rogers MRCVS,
Dublin, Ireland,
Advent, 2000

Rogers uses two technical terms in the text, "excess" and "deficiency", and this gave me a spontaneous continuation of the chapter. I will let Thoresen himself stand for the continuation. The reason for the following is the eagerness he showed many times to write this book himself during the course of our relationship. In my view, he would likely have achieved what would be inaccessible to all but a few international authorities within his field of research - a select minority of colleagues who have reached an understanding of his thinking and expression through a similar process as Rogers himself had to undergo in order to benefit from Thoresen´s writings.

I was first introduced to this natural eagerness when Thoresen was proofreading one of the other chapters. He could not restrain himself any longer, and thought it was high time to take action to correct one of mankind´s widespread perceptions of illness, a view which also I in my solidarity with the rest of mankind had conveyed to the readers. He therefore requested to add a few lines to my text, so that it was consistent with what he believes is the correct perception of what disease really is.

The "couple of lines", which became more than ten pages, did not fit into the chapter I had originally written, but in the chapter I have started on now Thoresen is by far the main character that I will not deny him column inches. I have produced an excerpt of what I myself understood of the ten pages, and I can guarantee that this sub-section, edited so that it should be understandable to most people, gives a good first impression of a way of thinking about wellbeing - health and disease - I believe everyone will benefit from familiarising themselves with this:

Health and disease

One can consider health and disease in several ways, and the definitions have also changed fundamentally over the years.

If one of the truly ancient cultures generally perceived health as a complex interaction between a healthy mind in a

41

healthy body (Greece in ancient times), or whether this only concerned the upper classes, I do not know, but this varied well with the different culture′s wealth. When the daily struggle to survive dies, one requires more of life than just being able to function physically. In medieval Europe the health of the average population were perceived mostly as the absence of physical illness, perhaps just to survive was characterised as being healthy. In our modern times, in rich western countries, the emphasis on health and wellness not only consists of the absence of disease symptoms, but also the positive elements as the opportunity to realise ones potential, balance, energy and last but not least *pleasure*.

These are more consistent with how we perceive health and illness within the complementary, *holistic* (wholeness-oriented) medicine – which in itself must be regarded as an excess phenomenon in our affluent society. Holistic medicine defines disease as *imbalance*, physical and/or mental, although this imbalance does not necessarily lead to external disease symptoms. Health can similarly be defined as *balance*.

But what is there to be balance?

• Formation must be in balance with breakdown.
• Sleep must be in balance with the waking state.
• Excretion must be in balance with absorption.

Besides a number of other processes.

If this balance is disturbed and somehow becomes unbalanced, especially in *deficiency*, then symptoms of disease will occur - first as imperceptible deviation in the psyche, in the mood, as acute or chronic changes in parts of the organism.

These symptoms occur, induced or created by ourselves to help the organism to cope with the occurred imbalance, thus inducing self-healing. A symptom is thus signs of an imbalance and occurs to alleviate the unbalanced process. If for example the kidneys does not work properly (in deficit), it must excreted more urine through the skin, and foul body odour occurs as a symptom, or it may be a dry eczema. This is to relieve the kidneys. We such not repress such symptoms, but instead help the kidneys to restore their original balance.

All the processes that governs life, must be balanced internally and externally in a finely tuned interaction. In order to help a sick organism with this we need to acquire as much insight into the character of the process as possible so that we can get a clear picture of the symptom.

Behind all manifestations of life lie processes. Everything in the organism are controlled and influenced by these - they balance or *control* each other in a system based on complex feedback mechanisms that either stimulate or *sedate* the processes to be controlled.

These feedback systems keep the processes in equilibrium. If this is out of balance then various aid mechanisms will come into effect, of both physical and behavioural nature, e.g.

- self-stimulation of acupuncture points
- activation of the ECIWO systems (a holistic system based on that in each part or each organ the whole organism can be recognised)
- regulation of the growth of hair, nails/hooves
- seeking medicinal plants (in modern times more in animals than humans)
- regulation of food intake
- compensatory processes that we experience as disease symptoms

The latter will make us feel weak and sick to a more or less degree, and if they do not help to restore energy balance, eventually chronic pathological changes occur. We must not understand the processes themselves as healthy or sick, similarly, a gun can not be described as either good or evil. Or as a Marxist said in the 70s: "A tractor can be either communist or capitalist."

Ordinarily we too easily perceive the processes that lead to disease, as "sick processes", and the processes that maintain health as "healthy processes".

Life (both plant and animal kingdom) has over the course of eons developed within the framework of a limited number of processes. These processes have adapted to numerous purposes, as in the different species shows up in different ways. For example, excretion of waste takes place in varying ways in fish, birds, plants and insects, but the process is still the same. Similarly, mental utterances appear in various forms of life in different ways. For example, properties such as affection or sexuality manifest itself in plants, fish and animals in ways that requires great insight and knowledge to recognise the common basic processes.

It is important to understand that life has not evolved sick processes - which in itself would have been pretty stupid. I will mention a few processes necessary for life, and what will happen when these processes are out of equilibrium either in excess or deficiency.

Examples of healthy processes:

1. The excretion of urine in the kidneys
2. Deposition of calcium, phosphorus and magnesium in the bones
3. Excretion of waste products in the colon, kidney and gall-bladder
4. Excretion and uptake of gases in the lungs

5. Hormone production in the glands

If these processes are excessively prominent, if they are acting in excess, they cause conditions that we experience as unhealthy and sickly:

1. Incontinence (bed-wetting)
2. Calcification
3. Diarrhoea
4. Dizziness
5. Nymphomania, pseudo pregnancy (imaginary pregnancy)

Note that the unhealthy and sickly conditions are set up in the same order as the healthy processes and are nothing more than the healthy processes in excess. This notion becomes even clearer if we set up this list once more, but now with examples of processes in deficiency:

1. Gout
2. Osteoporosis
3. Headache, constipation
4. Struggling for breath, anxiety
5. Disruption of the reproduction cycle

We may see from this that there are no processes which in themselves are sick. All processes are there for the preservation of life, it is only when processes are too strong or too weak that symptoms occur - in order to sedate or stimulate processes so that balance is restored.

All balanced processes sustain life. However, when significant psychological or physical stress causes unbalanced processes unpleasant and unwanted symptoms arise. Disease is an otherwise normal process that is either too much or too little – at the wrong place or at the wrong time.

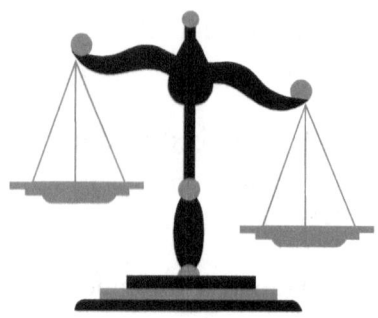

When it comes to cancer, the scientific medical research community has established that it is something that has gone wrong with our immune system and especially with the organism's ability to regulate the growth and shape it into functional cell structures. But here too, research has focused on the processes that goes wrong, with the result that we know much about what goes wrong in the immune system, which defences have been crashing, and nothing about what it takes to restore normal cell division in the organs or tissue structures where the cancer occurred.

This is because *cancer research's starting point is that the disease can not be cured by self healing or other natural methods* – that no one imagined that *reduced or destroyed "growth regulators" can be stimulated or brought back to normal functioning?* Or is it completely different reasons?

Could it be a factor that self-healing is free? Effective restoration of the organism's inherent ability to heal itself cannot be patented, a relationship that is demotivating for commercial initiated medical research - which overwhelmingly characterises the bulk of the research.

By making the general population healthier we will also strengthen the public finances, but at the same time this will lead to an enormous reduction of one of the rich countries' fastest growing and most lucrative industries, and [...].

I interrupt here because the relationship between economics and cancer treatment will be illustrated by Thoresen and especially his colleague Sergio Manzetti later in this book - referenced and supplemented by myself with my own reflections on the subject.

Thoresen medical views are still to be referenced, without my rewrites. This time it is not a correction of a prevalent misconception, as the previous was, on the contrary. This is a "new" field - new in the scientific sense, but with large, strong roots in traditional folk medicine - that Thoresen is spearheading, which becomes more widespread, even within the authorised medicine. It revolves around the concept of natural cancer treatment - this book´s continuation of the more ubiquitous term

Self-Healing

Self-healing occurs, at least occasionally, and although it is rare, it is nevertheless a reality and an opportunity for all of us. If only we could figure out how it can be triggered, how we can put it in function, which "button" to press...

The Catholic Church classifies it as *a miracle* when a person is healed from a seemingly incurable disease, without intervention by doctors or other healers.

The medical lexicon of Zetkin/Schaldach does not even mention the term.

Neither does Aschehougs major Norwegian lexicon.

On Google, there were nearly seven million hits for "self-healing", mainly descriptions within the category of alternative medicine.

In conventional medicine such events is characterised as not explainable events, chance, lies or patient self-deception or desire to get better. And if they occur within trials or patient evaluations, they are usually excluded from the experiment.

However, if self-healing really occurs, then the *possibility* of this must be present in the body. Not only in that person being healed, but within us all.

The truth is that self-healing occurs all the time, with each of us. All the time our body fights inflammation, bacteria, fungi and viruses and even *prions* (proteins that penetrate the cells, change the cell's proteins and allows diseases such as mad cow disease, scrapie and Creutzfeldt-Jacob syndrome). All the time potential cancer cells are disposed. It is only when this continuous self-healing deteriorates or fails, that disease occurs. If we ourselves, our own body, or other unknown factors can restart the self-healing, it is known in technical terms as *placebo*. If we are talking about serious disease, there are still many who will view it as a miracle.

Throughout my professional life I have been interested in exploring and mapping these self-healing processes, and then find ways to stimulate them to continued efforts if self-healing no longer is working *by itself*.

Based on my experience with self-healing, there are a number of factors that can restart it: psychological factors, artistic activities, music, plants and herbs, acupuncture, homeopathy, reflexology and osteopathy. Therefore, it is likely that multiple levels of information may lead to the self-healing systems.

Self-healing is within school medicine termed in many cases as placebo. Some have misunderstood the element of belief to mean that placebo is limited to that one *believes* one has recovered, that one only falsely *feel* healthy. Placebo has only occurred when, for unknown reasons, often because of a pervasive belief and conviction, one *truly has* recovered.

Most drug-trials are as follows: A group of patients receive the active medication and another group gets the placebo. The patients themselves do not know what they are receiving, but since they 're all sick, they hope that they get the real medication. Most commonly, a certain portion of both groups becomes healthy. And there are two factors that make them healthy: The medicine, and the placebo or self-healing. In the group receiving the real medication, for example, 66 % gets well. In the group receiving the placebo, 38% gets well. This means that 38% of the group receiving the real medication could have been cured by self-healing. We are then left with 28%, which probably has been cured by the drug. The pharmaceutical industry do not want to see that self-healing couriers the largest group of healing, because there is no money to make from self-healing.

Then this medication is produced, and all the patients who have this disease receive the new medication, and 66% are cured, and everyone is happy; the patients because they became healthy, the doctors because their patients are cured, and the pharmaceutical industry because they can sell their new medication.

But what if we instead could restart the self-healing? What percentage would then become healthy?

In sports medicine and osteopathy, we can find a parallel to self-healing. Normal muscle activity takes place like this: the brain sends impulses to the muscles through a nerve called "motor-neuron γ", which enables the muscle-spindles to contract. Another type of nerve fibre, Ia, feels the muscle-spindles contracting, and sends the information back to the brain. The brain continues this impulse to "motor neuron α", which then causes a contraction of the entire muscle.

When the muscle tightens, movements are blocked or fibroids are formed, the activity of "motor neuron γ" is increased in several muscle groups. The muscle-spindles are shortened, and proprioceptors send frequent signals that increase the tone of the muscles. These will be contracted and can no longer stretch. We get a permanent contraction, a state of disease.

Even with medication or physical therapy this condition can be difficult to reverse.

However, just by blocking the activity of the relevant nerves or stimulate one counteracting nerve, the whole condition may be removed, and healing occurs.

The same happens when we are sick. Our self-healing system has stalled. To restart self-healing it often requires nothing more than the right impulse in the right place and at the right time for the body to be able to take care of the problem.

All real healing is self-healing. While we can rectify mechanical defects and damage, something we can do methodically in physical- and chiropractic-therapy and by medical repair technology like surgery, it is only the body itself, our own self-healing systems, which can provide a full and lasting recovery.

Although surgery can correct mechanical damage and damage self-healing alone can not fix, surgery is completely dependent on an efficient self-healing. The organs the surgeon repairs and the wounds he inflicts on the body to get access cannot heal if your body does not let them heal.

oOo

Along this theme the Norwegian doctor Vilhelm Schjelderup touches in the preamble at the beginning of this chapter - the importance of *who* heals and the doctor's *intentions* -, the definitions of *disease* and *health*, and the inherent ability to *self-heal* are the very thread through Thoresen's professional life and therefore the major themes that can be linked most strongly to his biography.

50

5. Between Yin and Yang

Just as the opposing couple Yin and Yang are completely mutually dependent on each other for life to originate and evolve, our western culture's survival depends on us no longer to repel, but attract and cooperate with our opposites.

June 2012

Acupuncture behaviour is for those people who are born and raised in our Western or European culture, a mystery. For doctors and researchers it is unacceptable, while for patients receiving help for their health problems, this aid is usually sufficient to have a positive attitude towards the treatment method. In this context it is important to also achieve physicians' and researchers' acceptance that acupuncture actually works. By highlighting some of this medical tradition's historical background, I hope to open up to an understanding that acupuncture can have *an* effect on disease. To understand *how* acupuncture works, is a considerably more demanding project and must be left to those who give doctors and researchers training in this form of healing arts.

Before the technological revolution Europe had a very secluded place in the history of medicine. In all the millennia we can follow China back in history, however, we see the emergence of a sophisticated healing arts have been central to this national cultural development.

The fact that the majority of doctors and scientists in the probably still believe that acupuncture is not medical art, but something almost the opposite, I think is due to a combination of lack of knowledge and lack of tolerance. A steadily growing minority

52

believes that it is time to use all available knowledge about health, illness and healing for the benefit of a population in increasing need.

oOo

After reading the beginning of this chapter, which seriously touches his field, Thoresen is impatient to take the floor. He would rather have met this straight on, puzzled as to why he has never been understood - outside the inner circle of those who previously held assumptions in order to understand him and his research. This inner, but worldwide circuit consists of physicians from different cultural approaches to medicine and who have met under two basic assumptions: a holistic approach to people and the world, health and disease (holistic medicine), and extensive knowledge of the use of acupuncture, both the classical (Chinese) and the one which has been further developed in other parts of the world through the last century, especially in France. Acupuncture is constantly evolving thanks partly to Thoresen's work in Norway, which is known worldwide for many significant innovations and for developments adapted to the rapid changes in people's living conditions which have happened in his own lifetime.

Although I was quickly captivated by the principle of Thoresen's approach to the issue of the being of diseases and how to heal them, I understood very little when he would explain to me in detail what this was about. This is because the principles of acupuncture is very difficult to convey to someone who does not have insight into the perception of reality, especially the ones about the organisms, where the principles of acupuncture treatment in general come from.

I realised early on that it was important to convey this background knowledge from the well-known cause of many unnecessary "cultural clashes": that *he who understands, accepts,* while *he who do not understand, rejects.*

Even if Thoresen had no time to tell me about all the stages on his way into this new perception of reality, he answered at least some of the questions that otherwise would have required a study of

Chinese medicine at a high level in order to pass on to the readers something more than a superficial look. At the same time I could supplement with a prior knowledge of Asian culture, philosophy and religion which I had dedicated myself to in my younger days, in order to give a little insight into the long and strong academic traditions today's "modern" acupuncture is the result of.

I got a somewhat unorthodox introduction to Thoresen's views, like colleagues and students do, when once I was invited to one of his seminars to learn a little more about his work. Like the rest of the audience, I was taken aback when he began with the statement: "The first thing you must do is to forget traditional Chinese acupuncture!"

Was this a Zen Buddhist approach to rouse the audience from the dormant state they often bring with them into such an assembly - or a coquetry with the crowd?

My curiosity was satisfied when I later had the opportunity to have a little talk about what I had heard in the lecture.

- Did I really say it that strongly? It was not the intention. Not at all, I have great respect for most of what I know of ancient Chinese philosophy and science. But I have gained an increasing dislike to how the Chinese treat their philosophical traditions. Either they can not possibly have understood them fully, or they let them turn frigid - contrary to one of the pillars of Chinese philosophy: the duality of reality and its continuous dynamics as described in the doctrine of Yin and Yang.

Traditional Chinese Medicine (TCM), especially acupuncture, is unthinkable, impossible, without the existence of incessant flow and transformation. But while the Chinese themselves admire their cultural past, when philosophy was in dynamic development, the current TCM is increasingly entrenched in their old tracks. Do you know that the majority of the new developments within their own medical traditions, especially within acupuncture, are carried out in areas where acupuncture is a relatively newly acquired knowledge? Europe, especially France has long been a pioneer for both understanding and use of acupuncture in a way that promotes innovation and adaptation to the changes that have occurred over centuries in our organisms.

From a common acquaintance I knew he had been recognised in China as having found a number of new acupuncture points on horses and in the West also on dogs and humans. As an explanation for his introductory statement at the seminar he talks of contemporary Chinese people's conservatism.

- Excessive respect or lack of skills, what do I know, has not lead to the Chinese rectifying what has been wrong in the tradition - or that was right two thousand years ago, but is wrong today. Although constantly repeated experiences should show the Chinese, just as clearly as we see it from the outside, what does not work or is based on incorrect understanding.
- *Do you have any examples?*
- Many, but I will have to get into more technical descriptions. We can get back to this later after we have gone through some of the most important basic principles of acupuncture treatment.

What may be interesting in our context, is an equivalent stubbornness you have shown in the chapter "The riddle and the solution". It has taken 150 years of research on cancer symptoms, before anyone in recent years has begun to investigate the immune system to find the answer to the riddle.
- *You mentioned the doctrine of Yin and Yang. Is this an element of Chinese philosophy that can put us the on track to the differences in Western and Eastern mind-set?*
- Not only in the way of thinking, but also differences in assumptions for the very first philosophy we know. In ancient China it was no dominant priesthood who filtered the understanding of reality, while both in India and the Middle

East the clergy managed the truth. This caused the thinking and the conception of the world to be inextricably linked with religion in a form that was the premise of priesthood power throughout history.

- *When was the understanding of reality as a dynamic interacting togetherness created?*

- The duality appears in the Chinese history in a written tradition in the form of descriptions of the two primordial substances Yin and Yang. The earliest findings of the descriptions are dated to about twelve hundred years before Christ, but it is estimated that this philosophy and tales of Yin and Yang has been orally handed down long before this. Written records appear eight hundred years further back, before the founding of our culture's way of thinking, that Socrates, Plato and Aristotle, loosened the bonds between thinking and religion, and designed a philosophy based on knowledge and understanding, logic and reason. That which right up to the present time remains as the crucial difference, what distinguishes Chinese philosophy from other philosophies, are the dynamic interaction rather than antagonism and struggle. That which for Indians and Europeans will be dualism (the contradictions between heaven and earth, light and darkness, and so on), will in China be *duality* - a continuous, life-affirming interaction between Yin and Yang.

- *Does Yin and Yang represent the same contradictions as in dualism?*

- The same qualities, not as opposites, but as partners. Yin represents the earth and all that is dark, cold, deep, withering, wet and soft. Yang represents light, warmth, what is growing, high and hard. The Moon is Yin and the sun is Yang.

Before we end this conversation, I mention how I want to introduce the readers to the differences in the understanding of reality behind what has become Western and Eastern medicine, and I ask if he can consider which elements of Eastern philosophy that should be emphasised in such a context.

- Have you read Albert Schweitzer little yellow?
- *What?*
- His book on Eastern philosophical traditions. It was incidentally first published in Norwegian in 1972, which could be because he was in Oslo and received the Nobel Peace Prize in 1954. But it was written much earlier, around the outbreak of the war, during vigils in his tent in Lambaréné in Gabon. It was shortly after he had left his careers in Europe in theology and as a concert organist. After completing medical school, he followed the call he had received, and spent much of his life working to improve public health in Africa.
- *The little yellow?*
- The book is both small and thin and has a nice, bright yellow cover.

After returning home from the seminar, welcomed the first patients, taken pulse diagnoses and given them needles, he called me.

- The first time I was in China, I bought a copy of the latest English translation of the *I Ching* ("Book of Transformation"). You can borrow it and at least read the preface of psychologist Carl Gustav Jung. And - you must pick up a copy of an *Autobiography of a Yogi* by Paramahansa Yogananda. When you have gotten through this, you've got an idea about how crucial the differences of perceptions of reality between the East and the West are.

I had read Yogananda in my younger days and immediately agreed that he had succeeded in arousing interest and convey something to us so alien and incomprehensible as the eastern world-view and perception of reality. At the same time I realised that a great storyteller like him, with such good conditions - he also had many years of dedication of Western culture and the thinking behind it - needed nearly six hundred pages to induce a dawning understanding, That would not be easy to pass on here.

My ambition in the present book became reduced to appealing for tolerance of eastern worldview, to arouse interest in this type of culture and thought, and leave it up to readers to pursue any of the sources mentioned.

The western explanation of the distinction between oriental philosophy and worldview and our own is too often that our conclusions represent the truth, and that the opinions of others are the result of primitive superstition. In my view, it is the Europeans themselves who are enticed by naive belief - in the sense of a too strong belief. It is superstitious to take for granted that there is only one valid description of reality. It can be argued long and hard for such a statement, but scientifically considered, it is equally impossible to prove as different faith´s claims about gods´ objective existence.

It has been argued, suffered, tormented and countless wars fought throughout history based on the beliefs, opinions and management of Truth. In my work on this chapter, I have found that in the same way as one can judge gods and religions by their location in the ethical evolution - the gods should in my view have come a long way beyond us in moral understanding to deserve the name we have given them – we can judge the world´s many perceptions of reality. Not necessarily by their location within an ethical hierarchy, but how appropriate they have proved to us that carry them in our consciousness through generations and practicing their consequences in our lives and society.

When we judge what we are best served with, what gives us the most joy, peace, freedom, real prosperity and good health, we find that there is not necessarily an either or - Hindu or Christian, religious or knowledge seeker, shaman or surgeon - but both.

The long process that resulted in this book's creation has increased my own understanding of the importance of "Yes please, both!". Therefore I will by no means pit the Eastern culture and science against the West, but try to show the importance of mutual tolerance and its fruits: bridge building and cooperation for the common good.

Having said this, I must also emphasise the need for self-criticism, and that we, who are raised in a culture that always strenuously defended its eligibility by attacking others' beliefs and reality perceptions, should be especially vigilant for our own lack of humility. Is it not true that we in our culture are still so keen to maintain what we believe as the full and complete objective truth, that it may compromise the achievement of our work and our research's original goals? Did we stagnate in a kind of thought craze, so we judge everything that cannot be proven by our scientific methods as non- existent, as superstition or sham?

Behind this general topic and within this book's main theme, cancer research and cancer treatment, a specific question has increasingly manifested itself: Are the health authorities and the research community by routine and tradition become so bound by what is being considered as medical scientifically true and correct, that they without knowing have come to ignore or oppose strategies and therapies that can be at least as effective defences against cancer diseases as the authorised treatment?

Part II

Bridges and bridge-builders

6. The bridges

Like a bridge over troubled water, I will lay me down...

Paul Simon, 1969

When I became aware of the need for building bridges across the abyss that separates modern medicine from almost any other medicine - from our own medical history, natural medicine, and from other cultures medical traditions - I realised the need to establish a common bridge foundation on our side of the abyss. It's first about rethinking the concepts of *tolerance, understanding and empathy*, which in itself will lead us towards an attitude to other times and places' cultures where we realise that these *may* have come to an *equitable* understanding of reality as the one we in the West have today.

A first prerequisite to step out on one of the bridges I below will draw some sketches of, is reaching the basic level of scientific open-mindedness which means that it is not about being right and about fighting for our own beliefs or knowledge of power, but about cooperation.

oOo

Given my interest in *holistic thinking*[19] I sharpened my ears when Thoresen unexpectedly came with an admission that involved a real classic genuflection. And it was not a genuflection to anyone, but to someone many will see as his main potential adversary: Western and technological cancer research.

In my first apprenticeship of his newly developed method I had learned that the acupuncture needles are placed in different places, and that this is not related to the cancer type, but to the area where the cancer first occurred. To one of my very first "Why's" Thoresen said that it is this area's immune system he relates to, and this is what he stimulates with the needles[20]. My immediate next "why?" he dismissed by going a little deeper into an important consequence related to my first question:

- To be completely sure which treatment to choose, I am in many cases dependent on a pathologist using sophisticated laboratory equipment to have determined where the disease first occurred. It is not rare that the parent tumour is located somewhere other than where the symptom appears or has caused problems, and it will be crucial with a school medical analysis of a tissue sample to classify the type of cancer - before I can initiate a hundred per cent focused acupuncture treatment.

- *But I thought the immune system is the same for the whole body, and therefore only one way to stimulate this, regardless of the location in the body?*

- This has been the scientific perception until quite recently, but I can send you some references to recent discoveries about what might be termed the *partial immune system*[21]. This discovery should enhance the understanding of the mechanism of action in my method. Previously there has been no way to talk openly with generally trained doctors and cancer researchers on a partial immune system.

- *Is this based on an understanding of the immune system that has been developed within the acupuncture medicine?*

- To this I must answer both yes and no. That part of the immune system is linked to specific organs or parts of the body, a discovery I made almost thirty years ago, was at this time not something that was easy to talk openly about among acupuncturists either. But given that this is something I have both lectured and written extensively about in international relations, and it has been tested with good results through the cancer treatment method, one might say that there is an understanding that is currently under development in western acupuncture medicine.

oOo

If we raise our gaze, not much, but enough so that cancer treatment does not appear to be an isolated phenomenon, but one of many medical methods for our various ailments, one finds that it differs from the others as unsuitable for its medicinal purposes. The *only* cancer treatment we are offered - "only" in the sense that all other treatment given at special hospitals or cancer departments, is prohibited and punishable by law - has no measurable effect in relation to the treatments offered today for other deadly diseases[22]. In addition to this basic objection is that the treatment itself is so health disruptive that it inflicts on a large majority of the patients long-term or chronic injuries - in many cases permanent disability as a result. Cancer diseases appear to us as so terrible that they, more or less unconsciously, are also attributed the blame for the damage done by operations, radiation and chemotherapeutic drugs. What only a few acknowledge is that with treatment based on health restorative and life-giving care the majority of cancer patients would appear as healthy, at least much healthier than what is the case today, and they would generally through the disease have a much higher quality of life.

Here we encounter another misconception, one that probably has already led many readers to think that "without the health degrading treatment, the patient will face certain death." In the last part of the book, I will show that this notion is refuted by both statistics and new scientific studies. What I have termed as health restorative and life-giving treatment, are still too poorly documented, but this book's primary mission is to educate as many as possible that such treatment has been developed in Norway, and it has a healing effect that is far superior to all other known cancer treatment. At the same time I will show that this is already documented through controls in hospitals and tests in several of the world's most reputable laboratories within cancer research.

Prolonged under-communication of problems of cancer treatment with an exaggerated optimism about the future on cancer research's behalf has had a preservative effect and prevented that solutions have been sought in directions other than where authorised cancer research have been almost fruitless for many decades. There has been plenty of media coverage of encouraging research results and positive advance advertising for drugs that are being tested, but when it comes to *the bitter end* - how many people die, and how few people actually still survive the disease over time -, it turns out that this far, most of what has been launched in the market over the last fifty years, has had a limited effect. It is gratifying exception for some of the lesser-occurring cancers, but these give scarcely noticeable impact on the big cancer statistics.

This very little uplifting information is referenced here for the sake of this chapter's main subject: the need for change and particularly for bridge construction. I am far from alone in my concern over the lack of cooperation between the so-called *school-medical practitioners* and virtually everyone else, usually denoted by the term alternative practitioners. The need for changes in cancer treatment, especially a greater caution with the use of the most harmful measures, recently, in spring of 2013, about to come to the surface. They are not performed by critics of conventional medicine, but expressed from the inside of the "brain" of the Norwegian research community. In *Aftenposten* on the 23rd of April a researcher at the Norwegian Radium Hospital, Steinar Aamdal, and several of his colleagues express the same need to find replacements for the strong health degrading treatment.

However, there is a substantial difference from this book's basic ambition. Aamdal and his colleagues are all taking it for granted that such fundamental improvements in cancer treatment will come as a result of authorised cancer research alone.

But - as I have tried to show in chapter 3 ("The riddle and the solution"), it is a very big *BUT* in terms of whether the direction of cancer research selected for more than 100 years ago, could lead researchers closer to the goal. My hypothesis is that the wrong approach makes the fight against the symptoms always will come limping after a disease complex which has only been shown to grow and manifest a form of resistance that sometimes may resemble what is seen by excessive symptom treatment with antibiotics.

An increasing proportion of the population in the civilised part of the world die of cancer. In Norway, it's about 30 deaths every day, year after year, without delay and with a steady rise in recent decades, in which we have publicly available statistical material.

Apart from statistics for the final results (dead or still alive), there is little or nothing to find of research related to the authorised cancer treatment's medical consequences. Scientific understanding of the direct effects - large and physically traumatising operations, tissue damage and cancer-causing radioactive radiation and health damaging chemotherapeutic drugs - suggests that this is rarely about physical effects alone, but it often also has a mental disruptive effect. Among the deaths where cancer is given as cause of death on the death certificate, it is a diffuse but probably large number of which are directly related to hospital treatment and therefore only indirect bearing a relationship to the disease. This indication of how far astray the war against symptoms has led us, is an added emphasis on the need to replace the fight against cancer symptoms with *a natural and stimulating form of therapy that helps the body's own immune system to attack the disease by the root* - in short a treatment Thoresen's method so far is the best example of.

My main task is to show that the form of treatment Thoresen has developed and utilised through nearly 30 years of clinical practice, has a lot to offer conventional medicine through a joint collaboration. A few simple points can illustrate this thesis. We will start where the chapter began with Thoresen's admission of his need for modern technological diagnostic tools and continue the focus on the authorised treatment's weaknesses:

> • Without the help of authorised medicine the diagnosis by the acupuncturist/physician's pulse diagnosis in many cases will be far too inaccurate, which not only can make the treatment

ineffective but, in exceptional cases, also cause it to be counterproductive.

• Without the help of authorised medicine the monitoring and control of the further course of the disease will be deficient. The acupuncturist is dependent on modern X-ray and laboratory equipment as well as oncologists, radiology physicians and pathologist expertise to establish an optimal overall picture as a background for further processing.

• Without using a more effective treatment for healing it is indicated statistically that the results of cancer treatment at the hospital will remain so bad for the individual patient, it is a matter of time before it becomes widely known that to seek medical attention for the disease statistically gives about the same likelihood to aggravate the situation as to improve it.

• In addition, the authorised treatment gives only a limited predictability for a few patient groups regarding the further development of the disease. It is given no individual forecast based on the individual patient's health condition. This unpredictability is the result of the large distance between the cancer disease and the doctors' level of knowledge, due to the one-sided focus on the symptoms and lack of attention to the disease´s "origin" and its interaction with humans and life.

Predictability exists only in the later stage, to calculate *the residual life* - which really is more to be considered as a negative prediction based on that the hospital no longer has other than palliative care to offer. The prediction assumes namely that *the patient does not seek health restorative and life-giving strategies*, which in most cases will both extend and improve the remaining lifetime, in some cases even stop the disease[23].

• That the hospital's prognosis tools alone can not predict the individual cancer´s seemingly mysterious ways, they can be compensated by the acupuncturist's diagnostic tools – the pulse diagnosis. To the extent that the physician has learned the advanced part of the art of healing, it provides together with the hospital's technological tools one largely more reliable prediction as to the likelihood of whether the treatment will be effective - or whether it would be right and proper to modify the treatment.

The least inspiring part of the bridge-building is that the serious objections to the authorised treatment indicated above, must be made visible *to pave the way for the good news*: there is a solution if only the prestige is laid aside and bridge-building and cooperation are initiated.

Those who doubt the description of the lack of efficacy of the current cancer treatment, and trust in the periodically repeated messages about "the recent major advances in cancer research and cancer treatment", are referred to the documentation in the book's third and fourth parts. *It is emphasised that it is not referenced other than qualified cancer researchers, published studies or official statistical data from the Cancer Registry, Statistics Norway or equivalent qualified statistics from the EU or the U.S.*

oOo

The second bridge is described in the book's third part. It is already built. It may not be completely finished, but it has initially united two forms of research that is based on two completely different cultures. Specifically, this is about acupuncture research, through a scientific hypothesis, moved from the ancient Chinese traditional methods to molecular biological research laboratories in Norway, England and the United States.

Thoresen has been both the architect and the builder, but has received invaluable help bridging the gap between cultural contradictions - where molecular biologist Sergio Manzetti in a number of research laboratories has conducted experiments in order to test the credibility of Thoresen's hypothesis. Although I'm a complete amateur in both areas, the little knowledge I have been able to gain about acupuncture-theory and molecular biology - and Physiology -, has convinced me that Thoresen/Manzetti have begun a bridge that could carry considerable traffic of medical cultural exchanges.

68

Manzetti´s research opens unknown perspectives for a new generation of chemical medicine that combines ancient Eastern medical traditions with new Western technology. In itself this is a topic of a whole new book. What is being described here, however, is a kind of side effect of this research, a side effect that comprises of the bridge of understanding between the two disparate world-views. The difference in perception of reality has made it difficult, in many cases impossible, for scientific scholarly researchers to accept that acupuncture may be effective on other than "simple" disease symptoms, such as pain. The side effect of Thoresen and Manzetti´s research is that it allows for a general scientific understanding of how acupuncture affects the body's chemical processes. In addition, it has opened for the ability to repeat Manzetti´s laboratory methodology for any conceivable illness where acupuncture has an effect, thus establishing a medical scientific explained mechanism behind the individual treatment protocol - including the method Thoresen has designed to enable the organism to eliminate cancer. Due to that his treatment method is based on the analysis of the substances formed in the blood during the acupuncture treatment in the form of *peptides* that have not previously been detected, new drugs based on the synthesis of the same peptides, will be natural substances without toxic effects or other undesirable side effects.

A *peptide* is a chain of amino acids linked together. Several peptides can be folded and bound together and form proteins. When protein is broken down, peptides are also formed. In short, one can say that the difference between peptides and proteins is that the peptides are chains without any particular structure, while proteins are complete structures with a specific function. Some hormones such as insulin and neurotransmitters (signalling molecules in the nervous system) are peptides[24].

Thanks to Manzetti´s laboratory experiments, especially the described RNA- or mechanism experiment, anyone with medical training can understand how acupuncture works - and thus rationally accept that it actually works.

oOo

The third bridge is also built, albeit on a small scale, but nevertheless it is passable. In the first instance it will be used by either brave cancer-patients or patients that, after reading the description of this possibility in a summary of the patient's history later in the book, will understand that the combination I have chosen with the effective natural treatment and effective control and monitoring by a hospital is not dangerous to the extent folklore about cancer has instilled in us. That it is not *bravery* which is required, but *common sense* to try this solution first before initiating treatment with a major strain on the body, including the body's own, natural immune-system against cancer.

The summary of the patient-diary and the hospital records are referenced chronologically parallel with a summary of Thoresen/Manzetti´s laboratory research. Along with Manzetti´s own description of the cooperation, this bridgework constitute the core of the book's third section "Chi and chemistry".

oOo

The fourth bridge is *communication* - with the public and within the academic and political environments in which decisions are made about our future Public Health.

This is not a topic that requires any explanation. Instead I continue the work to convey what is relevant to gain knowledge about the new treatment method. Its effect is so far demonstrated by stopping many different forms of life-threatening cancers in dogs, horses and humans, and it is in the following explained in part and documented to an extent by the described laboratory research.

7. Meeting with Thoresen

70

Soon man will be his own
doctor and reattach the
limbs he once lost.

Novalis (1772-1801)

This could be the motto for
all doctors working in
awareness that the best they
can do for their patients, is
enhancing their inherent
capacity for self- healing.

Are Thoresen, July 2011

Finally, he was in place in my pavilion, on a temperate summer day
with the purpose of: jointly to gain insight into the areas of Thoresen's
life and work where subject and biography meet in a way that is
interesting for others than his immediate circle.

From poet and philosopher Novalis' optimistic prediction I
went further back, past the birth of Jesus and to the time and place it
was first foretold that there would be a transition from the mythic to
a rational age. I am not talking about religion or philosophy, but to
the earliest signs of animal welfare. From what I already knew about
Thoresen's first working experiences, it is the respect for animal
welfare rather than loyalty to employers that has remained on my
mind, and this is what I want him to tell us a bit more about.

One of the founders of Greek philosophy and mathematics,
Pythagoras (6th century BC), is among other things awarded credit
for making mathematics a separate item within the classical
philosophy, and to have established a philosophical school in the
Greek colony of Croton in southern Italy. The unusual with this
school was reportedly that it did not enrol students who ate meat.
Pythagoras' reason was, according to Plato, that people still standing
on the stage of development where they eat their friends, are not
sufficiently mature to receive the lessons (read: philosophy, from

71

Filos sofia = love of wisdom) Pythagoras would convey to his students.

It is currently impossible to know with certainty whether this is a historical fact or a legend. Regardless, the story witness of an awareness about animal self-worth in a time when men were still far from thinking of human rights and equality as fundamental values in the society construction. We are over half a millennium before the Sermon on the Mount, where a human life was not worth much compared to how we see it today. And, as we soon shall see, Pythagoras' way of thinking was far ahead of the thinking underlying the processing of slaughter in Norway until 1980.

> *- I've seen from your resume that you have a short career as a meat inspector. But you managed to at least make a major effort for the pigs before you left Bodø?*
> - Yes, mainly for the pigs but somewhat for the sheep as well. When I started with routine control at the slaughterhouses, I discovered quickly that the method for stunning that was used was not effective enough and this resulted in suffering. When I reported to the Ministry about this, the reply was: "who did I think I were, newly graduated from college wanting to overrule a method that all of my colleagues in the veterinary profession had accepted for years".
> *- Maybe not a totally unexpected reaction. Yet it must have been hard to prove this?*
> - To show that the pigs survived long after Norwegian veterinarians for years had considered them as dead, I gathered much information about the body´s reflexes, which gradually decline when unconscious and disappear completely when dead.
> *- What kind of reflexes?*
> - Like this...

Thoresen demonstrates the strongest body reflex we have, the classic strike below the knee - which in this case means that one of his legs flicks into the umbrella table and creates waves among the teacups.

- Sorry, but that was only one of the reflexes I tested on the pigs. Via this reflexes it was not hard to see that there was no more less life in the so-called stunned pigs than I have now showed you is in me. After referring to these examinations to a case manager in the Ministry, I received a letter saying that they would look at the regulations, and that in the meantime, I was free to choose another slaughter method.
- *Did you have an idea about what would work better?*
- A neck shot! I hired one of the earlier criminals in Bodø, which had solid experience with weapons. He was the perfect serial killer, and this worked perfectly as long as I worked there.
- *What happened when the Ministry had "looked" at the regulations?*
- Ha-ha, you beat me to it. New as I was, I had not yet learned that "looking", means just the opposite: they do not even bother to take a look at the regulations. And besides, if they had bothered to look and also realised the need for change, I know now that it can take years from someone deciding to change a regulation to "someone" actually doing it - assuming they skip the intermediary steps.
- *Which is...?*

It was clear that we touched a topic that stimulated Thoresen's well-known *respectlessness* - not for people mind you, but for very much of what they do - and I was curious about this intermediate stage of processing speed.

- ...that "we will think about it." This is a virtually perpetual stage, and whether the ministry does any thinking or not, is not really that significant, as it means that no action will be taken.
- *So nothing happened?*
- Of course not, and it was not until just before I moved from Bodø two years later, that I realised I had to do something. It

did not help the Norwegian sheep and pig population much if myself and my henchman...
- *The mass murderer?*

The attempt to follow up the light and humorous tone from my side was probably overlooked, because every time we approached purely technical issues and situations, the phlegmatic and laid-back attitude was quickly replaced by a sharpened pose. He continued without batting an eyelid.

> - ... the sharp shooter, yes - and that we together slaughtered a few hundred pigs and sheep in a more humane method than that used elsewhere in the country, did not do much for the big picture. Therefore I made an extensive documentation on the matter and stuffed three envelopes with copies addressed to Dagbladet (a national newspaper), NRK (a national TV channel) and the Attorney General my last weekend before the trip with the southbound Hurtigruten. Monday morning I called the Veterinary Director, told him what I had done and that I was going to mail the envelopes the following weekend if the regulations were not changed before the end of business hours Friday.
> - *Oh my! How did he react to that?*
> - Hard to say, but he dug deep and took charge of the matter, for the next Friday I received feedback that there was now new regulations. The next day I received another message as well, a phone-call, this time from one of the Ministry's lawyers. He appeared in the role as a kind of departmental prosecutor and told me that I had ended up on a list of undesirable people, and I could never expect to get a job in the ministry.

I reassured him that there probably were not any consequences either for the Ministry or me.

Thoresen had another cup of tea and told that his dismissal had probably irritated the ministerial actuator to an extent that he would make sure that the episode would have consequences for the rambunctious vet. At least Thoresen found no other explanation that his application for a State Veterinary job was not even being considered in Sandefjord, this according to one of the employees who were in the group which nominated candidates for the position.

Good thing he did not get the job, I thought, and then it was time to move on to the part of Thoresen's career, which is most interesting in our context.

> - When today has the answers, it's just as well that you ended as a private practitioner. But what you have talked about so far, was far from ending the conflict with the public health system. I have gained the understanding that academic success is not necessarily what stimulates collegial unity and cooperation. You have mentioned several episodes where reporting good treatment results only ended up with frustrations for you. I have especially noticed three events. The first thing I want you to describe, is when you in 2003 approached a Chief physician at the Norwegian Radium Hospital regarding the conduct of a clinical trial you wanted to perform on those of your patients who had cancer.
> - I first briefed him about the method I had developed to stimulate the body's inherent ability for self-healing. The purpose of this study was to investigate the possible relationships between stimulation of the self-healing and the development of cancer. I first encountered a positive attitude to my request and received detailed instructions on how I should set up and conduct the study.
> When I two years later sent him the results of the survey, I never got an answer.
> - How do you explain this break in communication?
> - I cannot explain it, but is thinking that the result of the study became a challenge for a researcher who has the specific notion that the treatment tradition they are

conducting is not only the best but the only one that has an effect on cancer.

- *You mean that the result was too good?*

- This was communicated very clearly by a female Chief physician at the hospital, which I later had a dialogue with. When I referred to the results of the study, she said: "This is too good to be true", and showed no interest in continuing the conversation.

- *From what I now know about you and your work in this field, it must be frustrating to be confronted with how those who manage consensus, already for many years have prevented, or at least greatly slowed, the prevalence of a method I have become convinced can help a large number of people who now die of the disease, especially since many patients have approached you as a last resort after being written off by the Norwegian Radium Hospital, and they are still alive today.*

It is almost lunchtime. Before we round off the insights into your career from the time before you started looking for the solution to cancer, I would however like to hear your own version of how the fine European statistics of liver problems in horses was completely destroyed after you started as a veterinarian.

- It sounds like the version of the story you have heard, have not included that I was first denied entry into this statistic, and that it therefore was allowed to be grossly misleading for more than twenty years. In comparison to what we just talked about, is that most of radically breaks with the prevailing notion are often either being denied or, in some cases, as in cancer treatment, prohibited.

The prelude to the example you mention, was that I through my own diagnosis method, a further development of the Chinese pulse diagnosis, discovered correlations between different disease symptoms in horses and an underlying liver problem. Because I've always been more concerned with identifying the true cause of disease - treat the evil from the root rather than treating the symptoms that ails the patients - I found that some muscular problems, allergies and also mental deficiencies was caused by an underlying and basic liver issue in more than half of the horses I examined. The reason why I was called out was mostly due to good racehorses without visible signs of disease or other problems began to lose their form. In those cases I noted a liver problem and dealt with this by using acupuncture, the horse usually very quickly got back to his usual spot on the result board.

- *How did the veterinary authorities react to your new observations?*

- They first urged me not to report my diagnosis of liver impairment, since this, as you mentioned, almost overnight had turned the statistics upside down in Norway. I was happy to be released from the reporting, but I got a little satisfaction when some years later a much more sensitive diagnostic form was developed in traditional veterinary medicine, which revealed that approximately 60% of horses have liver impairments. It corresponds to the number I constantly registered and treated.

- *That means that in the meantime, almost all horses with liver problems, that you have not had anything to do with, has been untreated?*

- Yes, a large number of good racehorses were ground to feed because liver problems eventually led to the horses simply became lame.

We eat lunch and talk loosely about the problems with being a participant and small cog in a large system one is constantly coming into conflict with and generally feel unwell in.

- I could bear to be a public veterinarian for long, within a social order which mass mutilated large groups of creatures that really should have been our friends, as Pythagoras reminds us. Instead they are objectified and denoted as *slaughter animals*.

I continue with the point on my agenda which is about how he, instead of enduring the daily challenges from colleagues and superiors got the freedom to perform his medical duties in exactly the direction he himself rated the best help for the patients.

> *- We have been talking a lot about that you neither felt at home within the established veterinary medicine nor in contact with the bureaucracy that controls it, largely due to the relationship that has evolved in our society with the so-called domestic animals.*
>
> > *Maybe you can tell us why it didn't become as you had first thought, that after the first years of discouraging experiences considered a fresh start with something completely different, but that you instead quickly developed a dedicated practice that gave you a living.*
>
> - It 's not often I judge life's phenomena as random, but the reason I did not become a house painter or farmer or applied myself to another earthy occupation, was one of the nicest chances I've been exposed to.
>
> *- It is customary to denote coincidences that lead to great changes, as fate or providential intervention. I thought maybe you had a tendency to see the world from such a basic attitude?*
>
> - Partially I am, and as a practitioner of holistic medicine, I have also trained an ability to see connections and meaning where most people see random coincidence. But when it comes to myself, I am careful to interpret phenomena.
>
> *- Why?*
>
> - It can easily lead to the wrong place, such as hubris - overconfidence - and to see oneself as more important than others. We've had enough of people throughout history who have seen themselves as God's chosen...

- ...and who you think has had such an opinion on the basis of ability or willingness to see connections where others see a chance or chaos?

- Yes, especially so. But this form of vision is, like most properties, something that can be trained, and it belongs as much to the trivialities world as the sacred. The reason that so few have this ability is that our cultural history for thousands of years has been a movement in the opposite direction and consistently cultivated the ability to see and study the details, which can best be done by isolating them from the whole, that is, by abstraction. Then the entirety disappears - it draws in a way back from the field of view and thus also from our interpretation of what we see. Those who throughout history have had special abilities to see unity and coherence have easily been exposed to either being elevated or stoned.

- It reminds me that when I asked one of your previous good neighbours to say something about how he perceived you, he managed after long reflection, not to think of anything other than to characterise you as "strange".

- Oh yes, - being different, I know a lot about. Ever since I was little, I realised that to understand or see something that none of the others saw or knew anything of could be both advantages and handicaps and I have not been particularly keen to disguise my oddities, but have constantly blurted out things I afterwards discovered that not everyone else has a relationship with or talks about.

I have tried to follow Aristotle's advice and choose the golden mean in this area. That is how I ended the oscillation between despair and hubris, and began to think about the special in the same way as the others think about the quite normal - perhaps with a little questioning addition: Why can't also the random be divine revelations of hitherto hidden relationships?

This statement gives meaning to my observations of how Thoresen always talk about even the most exceptional things in his life and practice with the same low tone and lightly smiling facial expression - in exactly the same way as he describes the everyday trivialities.

Still, I'm curious about the "coincidence" that meant that he remained a health worker and not a farmer or a house painter, and tracks him back to the topic.

- After Bodø, I gently started a clinic a couple of nights a week. I did not have many patients, and I began to think of completely different career choices. I did not actually have time for many thoughts on this before I was visited by a man who made sure that I soon had to extend the opening hours instead of advertising for patients or that I was free to paint houses.
- *How did he do it?*
- He had a particular health problem that no doctor or any hospital could help him with, and it was about to kill him. He could in fact not keep food down. Everything came up again, and so it had for more than two years. That I solved this problem in a simple way, gave me in a surprisingly short time so many new patients that I would not have had much time to spare for house painting.
- *Please tell us a little more about it.*
- It so happens that in Sandefjord there are many clubs of various kinds, particularly for gentlemen, and they have many members. My patient was the head of one of these clubs.
- *I see. He spoke openly at a meeting of the club that he had become healthy and how. And the first story about your good results spread from there onwards the local community.*

And what was the matter with him?
- He had an energy blockage in the leg that was due to a ruptured muscle two years earlier. The scar tissue formed in the area caused the blockage. That the stomach did not

function normally, was caused by scar tissue blocking the energy in what is described as the stomach-meridian and energetically is about conveying energy. The stomach is the central organ for processing and redistribution of the energy we provide the body via nutrients. When the stomach does not master the task of conveying energy to other parts of the organism, it rejected the food unprocessed.

One acupuncture treatment was enough to open the energy path, and he began to absorb nutrients normally again the same day.

- *By starting your own practice you had now solved the problem of poor communication or lack of understanding among your colleagues that you went your separate way. Your patients do not have any problems with the understanding as long as the treatment is working.*

- You are right in that I later in life have little experienced with incomprehension as a problem, although there have been a few more episodes than those you have mentioned today. Among physicians and veterinarians who use acupuncture in their practice, there is an extensive international network that I have contact with, and in Norway it is particularly in the horse-world that there is exclusively a positive attitude to my work methods. The results are the only thing that counts, and very few are concerned with why and how. No one has anything else to defend but his or her money, and they do not care about how acupuncture works - only that it works. There are often huge sums of money going one way or the other, and in this case the demand for acupuncture treatment is a reliable measure of its effect.

Within the public health system it is almost the opposite. Following custom or consensus is the main rule, what the majority subscribes to, and loyally follow regulations, finished recipes and then, possibly, look to the lessons learned as to what actually works over time. There is little room to use intuition, at least when it heads toward unconventional treatment or so-called "alternative therapies". I can and have practiced authorised medicine, and I know most alternative methods that have tradition and are widely used. However, I have for most health problems, whether it is horses, other animals or people, without comparison had the best results for my patients with the acupuncture method.

- You mentioned consensus in a way that makes me think of another rarely used word: paradigm - where it is so that before a so-called paradigm shift occurs, i.e. that new ground-breaking research leads to corresponding changes in the dominant thinking and practice, those representing consensus, shows stronger resistance to such changes.

- When reality is such that it is the elders who have the greatest influence on what at any time is consensus - and we know that the older people get, the more they resist change - is it a given that consensus is changing more slowly than knowledge we gained through research. Young scientists usually perform the unconventional research, seeking new paths when consensus is not good enough, with no respect for this kind of established tradition. This is how both large academic conflicts and a heavy backlog occur, which leads to us carrying ancient and little effective healing methods and medicines for too long. Especially difficult is it for cancer treatment because healthy competition is eliminated and all competitors to authorised cancer treatment are basically criminalised and threatened with fines or prison sentences. This monopoly situation increases inertia, even when it comes to account for pioneering research from within authorised medicine.

- You also mentioned that in the eighties it was to still so controversial to treat animals with acupuncture that it for your part led to a reaction from the Ministry.

- Yes, the matter ended there eventually, and the reaction from the Ministry was that I was required to adopt a written statement where I had to promise never to treat animals with so-called alternative treatment methods ever again.

- From what I understand, this was not a promise you kept for long?

- Not even for a moment. Loyalty to patients and their health is of course coming before loyalty to the bureaucracy. Moreover, this quirk from the Ministry soon became history.

- How so?

- After I settled down in Sandefjord, started my own clinic and had standing orders in the nation's racing (trotting) community, it was also noticed outside the racing community that I had good treatment results. One effect this had was that acupuncture now faced a more constructive attitude and two years after the special written agreement with the Ministry was asked to teach other veterinarians in some of the acupuncture techniques where the results had aroused special attention. I then sent a provocative letter to the Ministry where I asked for an exemption from the "ban", and was then told that I was relieved of my promise.

- One thing was recognition from outside the racing community, but it was still your work with horses that in a short period made you a sought-after lecturer and speaker in many countries and continents?

You have discovered new acupuncture points on horses, points that are now included in Chinese acupuncture, a subject I will return to later. Here I will ask about a couple of the "anecdotes", almost urban legends, being told about you, to see if you recognise yourself in them. The best one illustrates your international reputation in the racing community, and has a spectacular element where you are the protagonist in a private jet across the American continent. Along with two Indian vets you had been picked up by a wealthy Arab in his jet to treat a terminally ill trotter in Cincinnati.

- The Indians had nothing to do with the trotting horse, so there are probably two stories that have been linked together.

It was on one of my other trips I had the opportunity to receive an invitation from Indian colleagues to smoke with this Indian tribe's *shaman*, the local "medicine-man", which also managed the tribe's traditional religious ceremonies.
- *Do tell!*
- This was the initiation of a ritual that Indians want to preserve as a tradition, and therefore I can not tell you more than that afterwards they told me that this was the first time a white man had achieved a real insight into what this initiation is about.
- *Does secrecy has something to do with it?*
- Not really a stupid question. Most people do not understand why such rituals are guarded from the outside world and think it has to do with a kind of power trip of those who manage the secrets. The truth is that religious leaders where tradition is still alive and has not deteriorated into empty rituals and power strategies, has inherited an intuitive knowledge that the mind and thinking of people involved, affect the processes the rituals initiates. That face that few "whites" have been introduced in these tribal ceremonies, I see as a result of European culture having a tendency to invade other cultures, not only materially, but also with a disparaging attitude and not least with our highly developed scientifically scepticism, which can have a destructive impact on what it researches and dissects.
- *There is something called healthy scepticism...*
- There is also something called "there is a time and a place for everything" - and it's not unknown to Europeans that if scepticism is an important position in the natural sciences, humility and faith is what counts when it comes to religion. In this area you will not reach anything with scepticism than either blinding oneself or pushing the phenomenon being studied, out of sight - or both.
- *I am no stranger to that analysis or simply describing with limited terms what may turn out wrong, that only experience is what counts. Although I'm still interested in hearing more*

*about this, I will leave the peace pipe in peace for my
curiosity and go over to the other part of the story, the
reason you had been transported all this way by airplane.*

*According to the story I heard, it was one of the
sheikhs who runs Dubai, who had been told that you were a
speaker at a veterinary congress, and made contact with the
congress leadership to get you to look at one of the world's
most expensive racehorses.*

- He said he had paid $73 million for the horse and claimed
that it was the highest price paid for a horse at the time. This
was well into the 1990s, so he belonged to the group that
doctors like to refer to as so desperate that they even went to
alternative practitioners and quacks for help.

- *But you're no quack. After what I now have an
understanding of, acupuncture itself is an advanced form of
medical science. In addition to being fully trained in this
type of medicine you are fully trained in Western medicine.
It's news to me that veterinary education lies so close to
human medicine and that a veterinarian can almost be
equated with a doctor when it comes to all significant and
fundamental aspect of scientific medicine.*

- Yes, and my wording was probably closer to sarcasm than
a description of reality. Regardless, none of my medical
knowledge was of any help for the horse or the Sheikh. I
could, unfortunately, do no more than to euthanize it,
something that probably makes sure this story is not
something to include in your book.

- *Do not say that. Even if you could not save that horse, the
rest of the story is a curiosa underlining that you have in
many other cases succeeded where others have not been
able to help. That's the reason you were called, and it shows
how the rumour about your medical results have travelled
before you to places around the globe you had not yet
visited, and probably also to many places you still have not
been.*

- I could probably have been permitted to visit in Dubai, for even if the horse died; I have both at the time and later received an offer of keeping his other horses healthy.

- *Now I'm excited about what you have to say about the weirdest story I have heard about you, a story I've heard two different versions of, and therefore must be called a urban legend.*

- Now I became curious.

- *The essence of the story is that once you were called in to help a sick horse, where several people were present, including the horse's owner. While examining the horse, the owner suddenly got a serious ailment and collapsed, and when he was lying on the ground, you supposedly said something like: "Now the horse is healthy, and you can carry the owner inside, and I will take care of him afterwards."*

Is there any truth to this story, and what was it in this case that happened?

- Yes, it's more than a hint of truth in the story, even though it was not how it happened. This was in Berlin, and a female attorney owned the horse. The horse had an excess of energy, and she confirmed beforehand that I could direct this energy out through her.

- *This does not appear to be any recognised medical method?*

- There are many forms of energy exchange between animals and people who know each other, just think of the mutual affection between dogs and humans. Such so-called invisible ties that bind us together with other people and animals are actually ties, which in some cases can be utilised in cases of illness. However, this was so powerful that the lawyer fainted and remained unconscious for fifteen minutes, and when she awoke, she was so confused and unsatisfied with the situation that I instead of remuneration was promised a claim for damages.

It is actually funny you mention this story because I just gave a lecture at the Veterinary University about this method.

- *You are not controversial or at odds with your Norwegian colleagues anymore?*

- After having been non-existent for them for many years I surprisingly enough got an invitation again. But I am afraid that I probably once more went a little too fast and may have provoked them into putting me in a new quarantine. My problem is that I find it hard to be tactical, and since this is something I have practiced during many years with good results, I fell for the temptation.

- *This will for a general Norwegian appear as nonsense, but if I know you right, you have some sort of explanation for this variation of evocation or exorcism?*

I allow myself this characterisation of the phenomenon because Jesus had an opposite variation when he cast out a so-called evil spirit from a man and let it enter into some pigs nearby.

- You're absolutely right that it's not always easy to explain to patients or bystanders what is going on. I prefer a scientific description of such phenomena as energetic medicine does not see anything religious or supernatural in these processes, but place this safely within a slightly different scientific framework than the one we are taught to accept in the West. The background of understanding is not personified spirits, but energies in excess or deficiency. That energetic transfer between individuals is a completely natural process and can be described by how a yawn or a smile is contagious. Such processes are also possible to influence by acupuncture, not only between human beings but also between animals and their owners. Diagnostically it is often obvious to me, like in that event you mention, that the reason for an animal´s disease may be found in the owner. Then it can in some cases be more appropriate to reverse the process by treating the owner.

- How do you know it is about such transfers, and whom it will be most effective to treat?

- Here it is difficult to be absolutely specific. What I can say is that it's about a combination of intuition and through pulse diagnosis to verify whether intuition is correct. As in all forms of treatment, it's primarily about the results. This procedure has evolved over the years in such a way that intuition, diagnosis and efficacy is increasingly coinciding.

- This is still quite unclear to me.

- It is easier both to explain and understand such transfers of energy, and in particular the usefulness of them, when it comes to the treatment of infants. Between mother and child it is normally a particularly open and susceptible energy exchange. If this is something western science has not registered yet, it's at least easy logically inferred that it must be so: that the cut of the umbilical cord does not end the close connection, but that transmission channels move the center of gravity from the physical/spiritual toward the mental/energetic and then more and more towards the conscious and linguistically expressed.

Because children tend to be at least as afraid of my needles as they are for the dentist's drill, I tend to treat the child through the mother's energy system.

- How do you do it?

- After having diagnosed the child, I ask the mother to take the child on her lap. Then I treat her in the meridians and points I would have otherwise treated the child. An ear infection in children is a common health problem that I have good experience with treating this way.

Eventually I succeeded also to diagnose the child by feeling the mother's pulse.

- It's a long time since energy transfer was only about electric current through copper wires, so even one-sided materialistic minded ought to imagine forms of energy transfers that we in the West have not yet identified?

- We currently use wireless transmission of electricity, television and radio signals and laser, and can communicate over vast distances in the universe, so it's time to consider organic forms of energy transfers. It is after all the organisms that are always ahead of science and technology in terms of production and variety of forms of energy.

All researchers are working within their own "box", or knowledge horizon, which is both appropriate and useful for medical development - *within the same box*. It is when scientists speak with great authority about other medical researchers outside the box they have their knowledge from, that it becomes wrong. It is a recurring and unspeakable fruitless to always be confronted with claims by scientists with their specialised background that speaks confidently about what does *not exist* within other researchers' work field.

- *Based on your knowledge and experience you have postulated that the energetic impact of our capacity for self-healing causes changes in blood composition - which in turn leads to improvement of cancer symptoms. The fact that you actually deal with the blood and molecular biological studies of what happens in the blood of the cancer patients you treat, I have so far seen as a quantum leap. But now when you presented an image with the different boxes, it was obvious to me that it's probably not that easy to get brought in from the cold. As I see it, a conviction strengthened through many decades that no one other than the researcher within the established cancer research community will be able to achieve pioneering research in this field.*

- I never had the ambition to come in from the cold, as you call it. The medical basis is too different. The best I have hoped for with our laboratory research is to be understood. Getting Western medicine to recognise that acupuncture can have at least as large effect on physiological systems such as chemical medicine is essential. It is not enough to show *that* changes occur, it may still be explained away with magic and placebo effects. It is only when one can see how it works, through RNA (or mechanism) attempts, it becomes impossible to explain away that it's about intentional medical treatment which also functions as intended.

- *Your research partner, Sergio Manzetti, has explained this to me[25], so even if you do not have the money to lead the research towards a possible chemical medicine, you really have achieved what you describe as the main purpose of laboratory research.*

- It was probably naive to think that we could come in from the unknown and challenge the pharmaceutical giants in their own box, and if we had succeeded, it would possibly have been a side-track.

- *After becoming familiar with the effects of the acupuncture treatment I would go so far as to call it a dead end. Why spend hundreds of millions to develop a replica of a more natural process, and that in all probability would be an unnecessary and costly detour to an inferior treatment. Also, I think it would never have succeeded. The important thing was to build a bridge of understanding that the effect of acupuncture can be explained microbiological - not necessarily transform the method to a chemical copy. Among all the people I've talked to in the work of this book, is one that in a long life has had leadership responsibilities in the establishment of many large chemical-manufacturing companies around the world. The short version of his reaction to your ambitions in this field is that he was amused. Then my friend said that you would never get around these groups. He drew a parallel to how the oil industry has succeeded in halting or delaying competition in their main markets: gasoline and diesel engines in the world's car fleet, and pointed out that if you had been able to approach the market with a product with anything near the effect of acupuncture treatment, you would have threatened the investments the size of both the state budget and the oil fund. His conclusion was that any success with medical research would put you in a position that would create new and intractable challenges for you instead of solving the cancer problem.*

- The business world is a completely unknown field for me, so your friend can probably be right that we would be unprepared for what we could meet. But we already have acupuncture needles, not to mention a world where acupuncture is widely recognised and prevalent in large areas of modern medicine. Money is not needed, except for a small additional course for physicians who are already using acupuncture.

- *You use the word physician and not doctors?*

- In the big world there are often few and far between doctors who use acupuncture, while there may be a short distance between qualified acupuncturists. In most Western countries, however, it has become increasingly more doctors who practice acupuncture. Therefore there is no bold prediction that the route for this method of treatment must go through doctors - preferably in a hospital, so that it becomes part of an aggregate supply. There is of course an advantage for patients that expertise and technological equipment is in one place. My treatment is, as you've described earlier, entirely dependent on correct diagnosis by the hospital´s laboratory pathologist. Without such cooperation, I would not know what area of the partial immune system I should stimulate.

- *If we go back to yours and Manzetti's laboratory, it was originally an initiative from your side because we in the West generally only recognise what we as of today have been able to measure?*

- Exactly! As we get better at measuring processes in the blood with Western measurements and apparatus, or continue the work Sergio and others who have researched the relationship between acupuncture and Western understanding of the organism, has begun, it will show what I currently do, and apparently miraculously remove cancer symptoms, be obvious and based on publicly available knowledge.

Technological medicine is in its infancy, culturally considered, while there has been research on the Chinese *chi* and the Indian *prana* [both are terms for life energy - my note] for at least five thousand years. Because technologically developed measuring instruments have not been available for these millennia, scientists and doctors in the eastern tradition trained a sensitivity that also includes the qualitative aspects, not only the quantitative aspects that instruments can read. In that respect, an acupuncturist who master pulse diagnosis is in possession of a far more sophisticated measuring instrument than it is possible to produce technologically. A qualitative measurement presupposes a subject, something a "thing" can never be. In a scientific perspective will the fact that qualitative measurements may be different when several acupuncturists consider the result, be a serious weakness that are not taken into account. Contrary to what was the case before, where we had the so-called house doctor, who based most of his diagnosis and treatment to a large extent on his qualitative judgments, the modern medicine has not recognised the qualitative assessments value and for this reason not taken care of the intuition in a more targeted way by developing it along with the technological and chemical medicine. But I think probably many doctors still are physicians in the traditional sense, although it no longer is the basic element of Western medicine being discussed and researched.
- *Western medicine may get a lot for free by studying the acupuncturist sensitivity of the state of our energy system, not least thanks to the highly developed terminology that makes it possible to communicate the same sensitivity?*
- Eastern medicine´s perspective is that our life energy has both quantitative and qualitative aspects, and that we also have language and tools to manipulate this fundamental part of our living life. This has almost fallen completely out of

our language and our medicine because we on this entirely not insignificant area - ourselves - disregard what is not visible, while we are doing tremendous research on the invisible aspects of the things that are helpful to us in daily and professional life, such as radio, television, mobile phone, radar, sonar and so on. We have both language and tools for correcting the "life energy" if they do not work as they should. With the help of the tool acupuncture we can similarly both increase, decrease and control the energy of life and make a balance which means major qualitative changes for man, of his experience of his own body and his continued self-expression - repairs similar to those we in the West with a matter of course do, including the high-tech equipment at our hospital.

Thoresen inhales and look discreetly at his watch - he believes - and begins moving in the chair in a manner not to be mistaken. I do not have Thoresen for the whole day. But when I think of what I already had written in advance, and the amount of notes in front of me, I see that to complete a review of his career as an independent health worker will blow up the framework for my own work. Much of this will be indirectly treated elsewhere in the book, and the more biographical will have to wait until we sit with a straw hat and reminiscing backwards instead of now, where we are still gazing hopefully toward the future.

As for what could be the main theme for a more extensive biography, the years after he started his own practice in Sandefjord, I will here summarise by stating that Thoresen's creative approach to his subject has resulted in his development of acupuncture science now spread to a large number of countries. His theories, studies and treatment manuals have so far translated into English, German, French, Italian and Swedish, and it is planned a translation into Russian.

From these years, however, is one episode, which is neither an anecdote nor urban legend, which I must refer:

- Something I think many readers now would have asked you if they had the opportunity, is how you made the discovery that led you to help the large majority of the patients who have contacted you with a cancer disease.

- In 1983 I began to ponder over the possible links between cancer and the processes I read by pulse diagnosis. I saw a pattern, and it was logically enough connected with the energy that controls the part of our organism that *controls* growth. It is not necessarily something wrong with the *immune system* when cancer occurs, but with the body's own control of the cell growth. In Chinese acupuncture, there is something called the control cycle, but it has been in very little use both inside and outside China. This is what I decided to try out when the neighbour's dog got mammary cancer (breast cancer) that had spread to the lungs. I put the needle at the point I had arrived at intellectually would be the most effective to re-establish lost control of growth in that area, and I waited - like a hunter waiting for his prey.

He shifts position in the garden chair to a slightly forward position with an imaginary shotgun lying diagonally across the thighs.

- A month later the tumour was gone. And it never came back.

8. Eastern conceptions of our organism and life force. About the theory of acupuncture´s Chi

The one who understands, accepts, while he who do not understands, reject.

July 2013

If we should try to approach the traditional Chinese understanding of our organism, diseases and their healing, we should look at the elements of Chinese worldview that is most different from ours.

The most striking is that the Chinese clearly have a much greater respect for the past than we have. While we mostly judge most of what we did before, as quickly obsolete, as "medieval" or references to the stone age, the Chinese holds firmly on to the science they developed way back from the time before it was written down. One explanation we can find is in one of the first scientific books that has been preserved, the *I Ching* (oral tradition, recorded about 800 BC). The text collection covers the first science we know, and it describes the laws that determine *the changes* in nature, the universe and in humans, although it is about completely different forms of legality than those created for "the Western" universe.

Our science has an almost opposite point of origin because it primarily provides laws for what *does not change*, the constant laws of nature. Of course Western science describe change and movement, but within a static legality. This is an expedient "vehicle" for the early development of mechanics and electronics, but the cost of putting "earthly matter" in to servitude is a lack of understanding of and relationship with the dynamic and organic existence. What follows is naturally enough, the lack of understanding for other cultures where this gap between human and "matter" never occurred. The industrialisation of the east is a pure transfer from our culture and has *possibly* not lead to the same contradictions between biological/mechanical, organic/inorganic and static/dynamic reality as in the West.

From a Western point of view one can look at the differences in Western and Eastern understanding of reality as opposites that are mutually exclusive, so that one is right and the other wrong - or vice versa. This applies also to some extent the concept of "opposites". In the West opposites are often considered as being in conflict with each other, while in the East it is seen as interrelated and complementary to each other - as complementary, giving a perception of reality that is confident in its solid form, while it is in a slow, ceaseless flux and transformation.

The latter brings us into a mind-set that is distant to western logic, and which we may regard as paradoxical, that opposites that apparently mutually fight each other, in reality live peacefully side-by-side, creating infinity of new possibilities we can try and explore.

Seen in an overall perspective, the opposites that complement and cooperate with each other will cause a faster development towards something new and better functioning than those who break each other down. The latter we know from our science when a so-called paradigm shift cause a denial of the established facts as a result of being replaced by new ones.

I Ching describes the opposites that exist in the world in terms of a duality[26] consisting of the two basic principles of Yin and Yang[27]. It is not about antagonistic but complementary principles, which both contain the seeds of its opposite. Everything in the world is understood as an interaction between Yin and Yang. Nor are they absolute sizes: What in a given context is Yin, may in another be Yang. Hence, nature is not static, as something that can be defined and described once and for all. It is in constant transformation.

I Ching is subtitled "the book of transformation". Profoundly it can be viewed as a counterpart to our oldest academic textbooks, whether it is physics, biology, and so on, and it has until recently been

96

considered to have permanent validity. However, it is not too far for some "younger" (in mind-set and attitude towards research) western physicists to regard our own natural laws subjected to change, although some of the deeper transformations in nature and the laws that govern its expression, happens so slowly that we are not able to observe them within a lifetime or a limited cultural epoch.

It is here that also the traditional Chinese medicine, according to Thoresen, commits serious errors. In its cultivation of past masters and respect for what they came up with hundreds of years ago, Chinese medicine has in recent times overlooked the transformations in nature and also the probable changes in human nature that requires that medicine as a science must undergo similar transformations.

Where am *I*? Where are *we*? As children of our entire cultural history and not just the last centuries growing materialism, I will ask the following questions with regard to our *ego* or our *soul*: Is it me my surgeon sees when he operates in my head and peeks into my brain? Can he see me, where I rest unconscious under anaesthetics, awaiting consciousness and him going on medical rounds and saying he peeked into my head and seen how *I* in reality looks like? No, of course he cannot, we will respond, whether we are materialists who hunt for ourselves in genes and other cell structures, or we are convinced that our real identity does not have the form and content of the material or physical nature.

I am not writing this to convert anyone from a materialistic worldview, but for readers of this opinion to hopefully be able to recognise the *possibility* that what no one with certainty can know anything about, which is something different or more than is biologically surveyed, *may* be of non-perceptible and non-measurable form.

Without such open-mindedness it becomes difficult to understand acupuncture's central "area of operation" beyond the concept of energy.

And by all means: This "area" (in quotes because in our language we do not have a concept that covers this) that acupuncture and the acupuncturist relate to is not about the described *soul*, *ego* or *self*, but to open the understanding for what the Chinese in ancient times gave the name *Chi*.

In the middle of the organism, between the anatomy´s and the soul´s experiences, lies a mediating element that connects body and soul together and sustains both. Here it is no longer relevant to talk about smaller or larger, about duality´s static opposites, but of duality as movement and flow, stimulus, obstruction of flow, excess and deficiency.

The Chinese are disinterested in whether *Chi* is visible or not because they can *feel* it.

Chinese doctors and some Western therapists that uses acupuncture, have developed a sensitivity to feel/sense *Chi* through his medicine studies and later through his work in the same way as the sensitivity experienced physicians has for parts of our internal anatomy.

Chi is for acupuncturists, at least for some of them, as differentiated and nuanced as the external forms and colours are for us. Seeing *chi* in this way is probably also a contributing factor to the Western doctors who develops sensitivity and learn techniques to help facilitate life energy, can not imagine to stop this form of medicine.

In attempting to describe something I do not have special skills or training to deal with, I have concluded that it is easier for us who do not have this sensitivity; to approach an understanding of what *Chi* is when it is not present. My starting point, the way I'm used to seeing myself, is that the to me unknown *Chi* are, at least figuratively, between my experienced self and my physical body, which is the part of the organism that keeps me together as both subject and object and therefore an entire human, and ensuring that my body and soul is not whirring around the universe as separate parts. That *Chi* connects body and soul and sustains them both, is perhaps the reason why we in the West can best describe this area of ourselves as *life force or vitality*.

When it stops flowing life force in the organism, it is dead, and the whole dissolves. Anyone who has seen a dear one after he is dead, I think could have observed *Chi* through its absence: the remarkable difference between the expression in the face of a man who sleeps and when he is no longer alive.

Once in a remote antiquity people found out that monitoring and possibly help the flow of life force in the organism is the most effective way we can influence both the physical and non-physical parts of the organism. A larger number of physicians who are trained in both conventional medicine, classical Chinese acupuncture and other therapies, has concluded that for many diseases and ailments there are no other methods that give the doctor more excellent possibilities for an effective and fast treatment, such as "helping" the life force to run through us.

The challenge for Western medicine is that our medical school has neither given space or time for the vitality in the curriculum. This is again a result of that this traditional concept (constituting the principle of the direction that is called vitalism) has no place in modern science. Thus, it is also difficult to accept that influencing it, either by acupuncture or other methods, has no effect. To manipulate anything "imaginary" will not be particularly effective. Here I think we have arrived at the Achilles heel in relation to the difficulties of establishing constructive relations both with the official treatment regime and Norwegian research communities. The first step towards a dialogue think I might be to accept that we are not *just* a body of about 0.1 cubic meters of physical mass, but we have non-physical properties as well which are full-fledged parts of our organism, and which pervades and affects the physical body, both good and bad.

For many, the concept of energy will be a key. It takes energy to sustain life in a physical body, and it requires energy to experience something - to *be* the experiencer. A possible problem related to the concept of energy is that we in the West have a tendency to limit it to only include the properties of energy we can measure with the instruments we have so far developed. Then the existential aspect of life energy slips away. The subject, *being* energy, to live it, is not measurable, at least in quantitative terms.

After these reflections, and after reading Thoresen's definitions[28], I, as the western man I am, remain staring out of my window and I see the rest of life there, as a physical landscape, as an external world and an outer universe.

If I imagine looking the other way, east, or with eastern eyes, the direction is reversed. I look *inward* at living life, in what *is* the landscapes, the world and the universe.

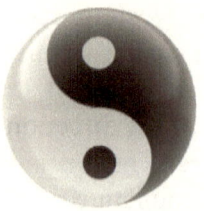

9. About the laboratory research

In the introduction to Part II (Chapter 6: "The bridges") a bridge was introduced that has united the two forms of research based on two completely different cultures. Specifically, this happened through a partnership between a veterinarian and clinical acupuncturist and a molecular biologist.

To lift up this cooperation from the personal level and into a form that involves the whole research institution is not done without an executive grip. Based on qualitative opposing viewpoints and diametrically opposite approaches to cancer as a medical phenomenon, structural changes offers major challenges.

The main basic contradiction is described in Chapter 3 ("The riddle and the solution"). It shall not be repeated here in any other way than by setting up some consequences of the difference between fighting the symptoms (tumours and metastases) and to stimulate the organism's own regulation of cell growth so that the symptoms disappear "by themselves" by self healing, usually lasting so that symptoms do not come back.

As I see it, it should however not be difficult for an unprejudiced "symptom researcher" to realise the benefit of either preventing a situation before symptoms become life-threatening, or to restore the organism's natural ability to sort and differentiate cell growth and division.

Although this means that one party unilaterally changes the angle of attack, and that further research be done on the body or organism's own terms, as these are revealed through Thoresen's work, the meeting can still take place in the middle of the bridge. To locate the meeting point we must return to the already outlined main contradiction: Natural Cancer Research sees the symptom as an important and basically friendly signal from the organism as the need for change. Authorised cancer research, however, consider the symptom exclusively as an enemy that should be combated. On the other hand, the overall trend in holistic medicine for turning its back on symptom treatment has the obvious weakness that it can easily overlook that there are a range of severe disease symptoms that threaten life and quality of life for millions of people, and where our health care system has been alone to develop lifesaving strategies.

For cancer, the situation is obviously the opposite. That this is not yet obvious to most people, I attribute to missing or misleading communication conveyed through the media. What follows in the third and fourth part of this book I think can transform disbelief to knowledge about a treatment I'm sure the majority of readers are still sceptical to - not least the question of whether it really keeps what this book claims.

oOo

After I was diagnosed in April 2007 I kept a diary that was going to be something my kids could get if it was going to go the way I considered was the most likely - before I started receiving the good news. When it became clear over the summer that I was not going to accept the offer of hospital care, E. and I planned a trip to the place we most of all wanted to visit again. The plan materialised in a fantastic week on the outskirts of Dubrovnik, where I on the balcony during the afternoon raised the level of ambition of the diary a notch and began to weave the notes I had in my laptop along with a travelogue from our vacation. The travelogue had "detours" to flashbacks from previous trips to the former Yugoslavia and more essayistic considerations relating to, among others, cancer issues.

About a month later I had a Thailand trip on my agenda. Because we still were counting the days we had together, E. became a part of what expanded into a new holiday and a new travelogue, characterised by even more distance to the personal aspect of the cancer problem.

My interest in simple mathematical models had moved from estimates of the likelihood of my own survival to an illustration of what I saw as a surprising new opportunity for relatively easy to check if it can be established so-called *significance* (highly likely) for

102

the effectiveness of Thoresen´s treatment method. This work was barely started in Dubrovnik.

A few years later it ended with a form of analysis that I think can supplement the very expensive method that today is the only one used to judge medications efficiency. I here quote the passages in the travelogue where this is the theme:

> "I've never been interested proving anything. What happens, happens, and whatever you do, you do. After I got sick and healthy again, however, I've become aware that there are situations where you do not get acceptance for what you do, if you do not also prove that what you are doing is the right thing to do. For example, if what you are doing is developing a new drug, you must prove that you have actually developed a new drug, and that it works as intended. If not, the health authorities put its foot down because you have not proven what you have done.
>
> Recently, I acquired some knowledge about this very special part of reality in which phenomena do not come into consideration as they are, until it is proven that they are. Otherwise they are nothing. In some cases, they must also be proved in a certain way to get recognition for what they are.
>
> In order to sell a new drug, the people who want to sell it, first have prove that a newly developed drug is effective, while not to be unreasonably dangerous. This is reassuring, how would it have been without such requirement for proof when we know how it can be - even with these requirements. An example of the latter is found by looking slightly behind the recently published statistics showing that the average use of medication for residents in Norwegian institutions for the elderly is eight different medications daily[29]. If we do not look too closely at reality and everyday life behind the numbers, it will be appropriate to automatically conclude that the elderly in institutions in Norway are plagued with a large number of health problems, perhaps as many as eight on average.

Fortunately it is not so. When we take a look behind the numbers that these statistics give us, it turns out that it really says something completely different. The statistics themselves have in fact never proven that each of the residents in the institutions are troubled by something close to on average eight diseases. On the other hand, statistics say nothing to the contrary, as we become aware of when we further examine conditions at the institutions.

Then we discover that the reality behind the statistics from the Norwegian nursing homes is that it basically does not have to be about more than a single health problem. The fact that patients are still served a menu of eight drugs, is due to the medical fact that the medication against this original issue, *on average*, has major side effects that creates new and so great medicine-induced health problems requiring a new medication, which in turn has major side effects requiring a new drug, which also has major side effects, and so on. This is how the importance of explaining the statistics from the concrete reality is stressed: what they *really* tell us - in this case that those who sell drugs to the population, have not provided satisfactory evidence that the drugs are not unreasonably dangerous, but on the contrary they are so dangerous that more medication is needed to remedy the damage they cause, which in turn causes a chain reaction of medicine use.

The defenders of frequent and widespread drug use might argue that the original health nuisance, that the patients first received medication for, is so serious that it justifies the subsequent chain reaction. The results reported by trained personnel and supervision of doctors at the institutions for the elderly in Norway that have attempted to reduce and in many cases completely eliminate the routine use of medicine to residents, clearly points in this direction. These experiments have in common *that residents consistently have been healthier and more awake, enterprising and satisfied than they were when they ate an average of eight different medications daily."*

Of the drugs that are considered to be the most harmful, most are in the long list of drugs used in the treatment of various cancer diseases. Along with radiotherapy and surgery these medications cause such a large burden on patients that some doctors have begun to ask whether many cancer patients would have survived at least as long and had a better life ending without these medications. Here we are possibly in front of a monstrous dilemma. It appears that those making the decisions have closed both their and our eyes to the problem.

The dilemma can be expressed as follows: *Given that some are cured by the treatment, we can not stop giving the medication even if we are aware that other dies from it.*

The only way out of the dilemma is the development of a type of medicine that not only claims to be harmless under the circumstances, but in practice also turns out to be harmless. In the example of the elders mentioned above, it appears that many approved drugs are so dangerous that they lead to severe over medication.

To find out if the problem of dangerous medication has any connection with what kind of evidence is required by the pharmaceutical industry with regard to the drug effects, one must look at how drugs are approved by the government. Maybe this will also reveal adverse effects other than that many of the elders in our communities wither and die before their time really is up.

First some general considerations regarding the documentation of drug's effects.

Research confirms itself and its relevance through two main forms of evidence: *universal* or *pure probability calculation* and *statistical probability calculation* (statistical significance). The first method requires that all data on which the calculations are done are reliable, and that there are only a few and insignificant, preferably no one, known sources of error. An example of this form of probability calculation is that a substance is tested in a recognised laboratory by adding it to a cancer culture *in vitro* (in glass test tubes, petri dishes, and so on). If the preparation has an effect on cancer cells, for example, kills them, it established a pure probability that it will work the same way if we repeat the experiment - in the same laboratory, in other laboratories or also adds the substance to the same type of cancer cells under other conditions. The transfer to other conditions, such as cancer cells in an organism, has an uncertainty factor that reduces the probability so much that we must carry out the experiment in a similar organism to obtain pure probability. If you want to create probability that the product also has an effect on people in general, not just the test person, statistical probability is required - that many have to participate in the experiment.

Testing of cancer medicine occurs in the first stage by pure probability calculation (laboratory tests) and followed by statistical probability calculation (animal and human trials). Human trials are conducted on large groups, of more than a hundred people, and they include a control group receiving the inactive medicine without any of the participants knowing who gets what. This last will by a statistically calculated results eliminate that the placebo becomes an underlying uncertainty in the trial. The experiment is only successful if there is a *significant*, a substantial and predefined difference in disease progression in those who have received the active medicine, and those who have been given "sugar pills".

For some serious diseases, like cancer, ethical constraints make it impossible to implement "real" statistical probability calculations on people. And this is important: Because it is ethically reprehensible to postpone or cancel an authorised treatment for cancer for the sake of such a trial, we know nothing about how the increasing flood of new, expensive cancer drugs in reality acts on the entire group of cancer patients. What we will know is the *statistical most likely impact on cancer patients who have not been cured by authorised treatment, and who are no longer offered authorised treatment*. It is only this group, that is, *terminal* patients, who for ethical reasons are offered a place to participate in the trial of new anticancer drugs.

Putting it bluntly, we can put it like this for ethical reasons, no new cancer drugs are tested on the group of patients who are the real target audience for the medicine.

Natural follow-up questions are:

- Who is aware of this?
- Who is not aware of this of those who should be?
- Is additional precaution taken for the cancer patients receiving medication not tested in that category of patients they are located in?
- Is this something cancer patients are or may be advised of before they must decide whether to try drugs?
- Or is this something only scientists/doctors/Norwegian Medicines Control Authorities are aware of, and patients know nothing about, because their judgment is not trusted enough to assess whether they should take the risk or not to take the most dangerous and perhaps least proven medicines on the market?

In addition to the ethical problem those patients who are subjected to the trials, will be so strongly weakened by the disease[30] and so strongly influenced by the treatment that the results of the trial are not directly transferable to humans in reverse mode: those which are in an early phase of the disease and with normal functioning organs and immune system. These patients constitute by far the largest group of those cancer patients who have recently been diagnosed and therefore in many cases represent the medicine's biggest target if it is approved through trial.

This is not just a theoretical problem, but also an issue that has been shown to actually have dramatic consequences for cancer patients. The claim here about the fatal effects of anticancer drugs that have not been tested in the intended patient population are described and documented in Chapter 10 (" Back to the patient diary. An epitome").

In such situations, the figures are not to be trusted. Statistical confirmation of the effect on terminal patients may be worthless and in many cases misleading in terms of dangerous side effects for cancer patients in the early stage - because *it is not checked whether the drug can have dangerous side effects in this patient group*. Anyone that deals with numbers in their subject of specialisation will immediately see that the numbers seeming credibility in such cases is used in a way that hides the real underlying truth.

One who understands the numbers seeming absoluteness will see that they in this case might mislead patients into believing that the medication they are offered, are thoroughly tested on patients who are in a similar situation as themselves, and that the statistics they may be presented, are valid for them, while this is not at all the case.

oOo

When I got cancer, I had not much knowledge about this disease. I knew what most knew, those who had not had it in their lives - in their immediate circle or in their own body.

In the meantime, three of the closest in my wife's and my family had cancer. One survived, while the other two died from the disease. This ratio, one to two, is possibly reflecting my own odds. This assumption is more a feeling; based on facial expressions and ambiguous statements by the professionals I have so far had contact with, than the result of my interest in *living figures*[31]. This part of the statistics I had not had any special interest in. The odds were bad anyway for this cancer type, and especially bad in my case because of the size of the tumour[32].

After the disease came into our family, the interest for both authorised and alternative cancer research grew naturally enough. Thanks to the insight that reinforced interest eventually gave me, I discovered a serious weakness in the area of cancer research that involves the testing of potential medications. Now, a month later, I'm still amazed at how it can be possible that something as obvious for so long have been so well hidden.

I think I already the night after this discovery had my first thoughts about a story where a scientist set out to prove that there is a way to avoid this weakness in cancer research, more accurately

108

expressed as a fatal mistake, that for decades has been committed prior to the approval of new cancer drugs. The error is due to that, for some reason, it is embodied an absolute requirement of so-called *statistical significance* before a drug is approved for general use, that it is a statistical probability that it really does have the intended effect on the group(s) of patients it has been developed for.

The requirement is fully understandable if it had been fully possible to comply with it. It is not. Such evidence is in fact completely unethical to establish by the trials of most cancer drugs because it assumes that a large group of patients, the so-called control group not offered the existing cancer treatment, which for most cancer patients would be an unacceptable health risk. Therefore, the testing is limited to a group of cancer patients where one claims that there is no risk to be in the control group. To end up in the control group means that one is given an inactive preparation of the same shape and colour as the real drug. The postulate "that there is no risk", is derived from another postulate, namely that all patients in this group regardless are going to die. In other words, the risk for the patients in the control group, is that they do not get to enjoy any life-prolonging effect of the real medication.

In the story that began to take shape in my head, *my* researcher discovered this weakness in cancer research. When she claimed to have developed a medicine that could cure cancer in all stages of the disease, provided that no tumour or cancer treatment had given fatal damage to the organism, she suggested introducing a new practice for this type of medication. One should maintain the general requirement to test the drug on the groups it was intended for, but forgo the requirement of statistical probability calculation (significance). The most obvious is switching to a method here designated as *ordinary probability calculation*.

The medication the researcher had developed, had little or no effect on patients who had undergone chemotherapy. It must be used at an early stage of the disease, before patients eventually had used chemotherapy. Because of chemotherapy's disruptive effects on our immune system the medication failed to improve or restore the body's natural defences against cancer enough that the disease was retarded. Consequently, it would be futile to try the medication on this patient group - *the only group of patients which is currently regarded as ethically justifiable to use the testing method in which a control group is given the placebo.*

The researcher suggested a trial on patients who had not yet received chemotherapy, but without a control group with the placebo. This would eliminate the ethical issue, but this deviation from the predominant method for trials was denied. The only remaining possibility for an effective testing on humans without breaking the current ethical guidelines or Norwegian law, was that the researcher induced cancer in herself - in the same way as it is done in mouse experiments - in order to verify whether the product would have any impact on the further course of the disease.

Since the decision is mine, in my own story, I equip the scientist with an extraordinary courage, and she conducts a trial of the drug on herself after having induced cancer in herself where it was easiest to reach, namely in one breast. The experiment was successful. The tumour she had operated in first grew normally, but after she took her own medicine, the tumour stopped to grow. Biopsies taken some weeks later showed that the cancer cells no longer had the ability to infiltrate other tissues or organs. Expressed in a more folksy way, the cancer cells were disarmed, and the tumour was changed from malignant to benign.

Although her cancer had stagnated and changed to a harmless lump in the breast, the established medical research would not admit this change had anything to do with her medication. Her fellow researchers classified this research result as anecdotal healing. It did not help the researcher to claim that it was a planned effect caused by the medication she had injected into the tumour, since the superior researchers claimed that the effect was due to an accidental coincidence. They believed that this remarkable healing just as easily could have occurred without injecting the medication. Therefore, we must establish statistical significance, it was said, to eliminate that it may have been a matter of chance rather than anecdotal healing.

110

Her argument that an attempt to establish statistical significance for ethical reasons was impossible and did not make an impression.

The researcher was no further forward.

Anecdotal healing has been given this common name because the cure of cancer with no known detectable cause are so rare that they can not be classified or differentiated in other, separate designations. The scientist, who, not unlike myself, is concerned with living figures, did not give up. Instead, she made some thoughts about the probability that anecdotal healing occurs within a given period. The given time in this case will be from when the disease is diagnosed, and the selected treatment can begin, a period that would normally be at least a month because it requires a series of tests and examinations before a decision can be made about the right course of treatment. If anecdotal healing had occurred frequently, for example more frequently than one in a thousand cases, they should have been captured as a statistically known factor as in that the improvement would precede treatment and make it superfluous. For comparison, corresponding to a frequency of such degree - more often than one in a thousand - one of the categories for the drug's side effects are shown in the overview (PDR) of the medicines sold in Norway, *Felleskatalogen*. If there had been improvement in this period (one month) for more than one thousand newly diagnosed patients, this should have been in the statistics as x number per thousand of the total number of diagnosed cancer cases. The researcher therefore believed to be on safe ground when she concluded that such a probability might be less than one in a thousand.

On the other hand: The few cases we are talking about, is impossible to estimate in that they obviously are so rare that no one has seen it as an exciting challenge to figure out why some are cured before they start treatment. In the researcher's eyes this would be the only explanation for why rare spontaneous healing had never been regarded as anything but either misdiagnosis or other accidental and non-scientific cause, such as a miracle - or just an anecdotal healing. For this reason they have never been subject to scientific research, but they should make for very interesting cases of natural healing or *self healing although it is* admittedly rare.

After these reflections on why her research results were dismissed, she was left with the statistical fact that it's a probability of the order of one to a thousand or less that her healing was caused by anecdotal healing and not by the medication she had developed.

PDR classifies adverse events occurring in lower numbers than one in a thousand as *rare* - so rare that they are not always included in the list of side effects. It does not mean they can not occur, just as the scientist probability calculation can not completely rule out that there was an anecdotal healing and not the product that cured her. In this the researcher had to admit that the senior scientists were correct, but it did not prevent that she still thought to justify the claim that a *pure probability calculation* will provide a reliable indication of whether a medication is effective, and that such a calculation would be an acceptable alternative to *statistical probability* where it is not ethically justifiable to use this method. She also drew the conclusion that in the case of cancer diseases in particular, a pure probability calculation applied *to the particular patient population* to be a far better option than the statistical probability (significance) used *on another group of patients than the medication is primarily intended for.*

So far, after conducting the experiment on herself, the researcher could with a basis for a mathematical calculation show a likelihood of a thousand to one that the medication would heal the particular cancer. This was as said not satisfactory to her older and more experienced colleagues. She therefore decided to repeat the experiment on herself. It gave the same result as last time. Before one month had passed, MRI showed that the tumour had stopped growing, and biopsy showed that the cancer cells no longer had the characteristics required to be termed cancer cells.

Naturally enough, this impressed everyone who heard about the experiment. With one exception. Her superiors in the research institution where she works hardly raised an eyebrow when they were presented with her latest research. One plus one is two, they said, and two are not much more than one when it comes to establishing statistical significance. They had not heard of the concept of universal or pure probability and what the difference between those involved (naturally enough, since it was she who had made them), and they were not interested in hearing about it when it was presented by a junior researcher and not a superior authority. Nor did any of them express that they had taken in the actual outcome: she had probably been cured once again after taking the medication she had developed. Non of her fellow researchers commented on this.

Naturally enough, the researcher became very disappointed. She had become a researcher primarily based on the notion that research institutions' primary mission is to safeguard and secure knowledge, including knowledge of the yet unexplored. She saw it as crucial that new and potentially useful information to society are well taken care of and thoroughly researched before discarded as uninteresting.

I almost take for granted that most non-scientists have the same confidence in the research institutions that this researcher had originally. For *it is Askeladden's (the Ashlad) curiosity and openness to phenomena and not Per and Pål's besser-wisser scepticism that is the researching ideal* (Norwegian folk-lore).

oOo

Before I put away the anecdote, I will present a slightly kinder version with a happy ending. I imagine that the story's brave scientist really has succeeded in opening research colleagues and health authorities' eyes to the ethical dilemma that it is impossible to establish the relevant statistical significance prior to the approval of drugs used in cancer patients in the early stages of the disease. Even though it is proven that dying cancer patients receive a positive effect from a drug under testing, this does not necessarily mean that it can be used on yet untreated patients. In my view, it is an obvious fallacy in relation to the purpose of proving the drug's effects that it should have been obvious to the researcher's colleagues to also see this fallacy. But what do they do when they are faced with this embarrassing dilemma?

Yes, the ones that in the previous version of the story who were the bad ones, have now become kind and realise that in this case rule-bound bureaucracy should not apply, but a pragmatic approach to get out of the untenable situation. Here we must use common sense.

The most suitable means that reason has at its disposal to arrive at a certain knowledge in such cases is to make probability calculations. The alternative to *statistical probability calculation* is as I said a *pure probability calculation*. Our new hero gets an exemption from the health authorities from the absolute requirement of statistical significance and presents the results obtained for a mathematician.

Having been told the anecdote about the brave scientist and heard her research colleagues' conclusion the mathematician is protesting loudly against that "one plus one" in this case is "two", and points out that it must be multiplied and not added in this case.

> - A simple experiment multiplied by an identical and repeated experiment with the same results will lead to an exponential increase of the probability that the result is obtained as a result of a plan and not by coincidence. For example, an experiment in which the probability of achieving a particular result by chance is one-tenth, indicate that two identical results lessens the chance that this could have occurred by chance, to one in a hundred. Scientifically considered, this means that the uncertainty is approximately zero, and that in this case we can almost determine that healing is due to the medication.
> - *Before we asked you to help understand this point, we have thanks to the available information on the incidence of so-called anecdotal cures concluded that they must be rarer than one in a thousand. Had they occurred very frequently, we would have caught them up in our statistics - something we have not done.*

- Then the probability will rise to a million to one and the uncertainty definitely has lapsed - unless you mean placebo will have an impact on cancer tumours.

- *Cancer researchers have always disregarded that. What if I add that both times the healing happened shortly after the treatment, i.e. within a limited, defined period of let's say one month?*

- There will be an estimated tenfold unlikelihood that we are dealing with anecdotal healing. We are as close to a figure of eight zeros to one in favour of the probability that the reason for the improvement was treatment, not that it happened by chance.

oOo

The foregoing is not "just" an anecdote or imagination. The reality it refers to will be described in Chapter 10 ("Back to the patient diary. An epitome")[33]. The attentive reader will realise the reason the anecdote was born.

If this still appears to be an enigma, the final solution will come – like in a crime novel - in the book's last and fourth part.

Part III

Chi and Chemistry

10. Back to the patient diary. An epitome

2007

Colonoscopy and subsequent rectoscopy left no doubt that my problem was not a harmless cyst, which I had little hope for, but a malignant tumour the size of something between a plum and a tangerine according to my GP Bard Nome in Sandefjord.

I declined the offer to take a biopsy of the tumour of fear of spreading cancer cells by the bloodstream. At the same time I was afraid to weaken the body's immune system by taking chemo - though this possibly would have reduced the risk of spreading, which a surgeon probably eluded when he denied that biopsy of a malignant tumour would lead to a risk of spreading.

The day after the diagnosis, 18th of April, Thoresen gave me a targeted stimulation of the body's capacity for self- healing based on the hospital's diagnosis of where the cancer had first occurred. On the basis of acupuncture's premier diagnostic tool, the pulse diagnosis, Thoresen confirmed two months later that the treatment had affected the body's processes or *energy balance* (a more popular mode of expression than an acupuncturist will use). MRI and CT showed no metastasis or spread to other organs. After what I knew about this newly developed acupuncture method's mode of action, I was no longer so scared to take a biopsy, and after continued pressure from the hospital I now accepted this - not least so as not to appear as a problematic patient.

An experienced and reputable gastrologist, Geir Haarberg, then took three biopsies of the tumour and was the same day accused by the pathologist to have missed or hit peripheral in the tumour. Haarberg confirmed by phone, on my direct question, that he was such an experienced surgeon that he mastered this task, and he denied that he could have missed the tumour. The cause of the pathologist accusation was that he found cancer cells without cancer properties, described to me by Nome, who translated the Latin, to "cancer, but not cancer" - later explained by the oncologist Gustafson as "non-malignant cells". She explained this as cancer cells without metastatic properties, that is, that do not have the ability to infiltrate the surrounding tissues or other organs, which, as I understand it really was not cancer.

Doctors at the Norwegian Radium Hospital claimed that there had to be malignant cells in the tumour, they just had not found any yet. My own conclusion was that the pathologist, oncologist and other doctors were faced with a phenomenon, which in their opinion could not happen in a case like mine. For them, the explanation was that Haarberg had missed with the biopsy. Except from Gustafson and Nome, the doctors strategy in the time that followed, was to "scare me" to the operating table, which I experienced as the opposite of my own method to combat the disease. I was later told by a surgeon at the Norwegian Radium Hospital that there is such a general strategy that doctors should abide by in case the patient does not follow their treatment advice. In my case it simply consisted of them constantly warning me that I risked death if I did not follow their treatment advice. This seemed highly psychologically destructive to me and worked against the treatment I had actually chosen.

I deliberately chose never to give any advance information to Thoresen about my condition or the results of the checks at the hospital, as I was curious if he could read the development of the disease by pulse diagnosis. There was always agreement between the pulse diagnosis and the controls in the hospital, and my mental lows after visits to the Norwegian Radium Hospital this summer was read as new disturbances in the energy balance. In my assessment his treatment significantly consisted on restoring my inner strength. A new pulse diagnosis after the summer showed that the intended change was achieved.

After hard pressure from doctors both in Vestfold Hospital and the Radium Hospital I once more gave into the pressure and took new biopsies. Another experienced surgeon, Jens Marius Næsgaard, took three deep biopsies, so deep that I got a violent bleeding after I got home, and for an hour feared I would die of blood loss instead of cancer. I fell asleep or passed out before I had decided to call an ambulance and destiny would have it that the bleeding must have stopped just after I "disappeared". When I woke up in the morning there was no more blood collected in the intestine.

The pathologist once again found only the same type of benign tumour cells. New MRI showed no growth in the tumour, which should be a strong circumstantial evidence that the total of six biopsies that were taken from the tumour, and all showed the same, was properly conducted. They all confirmed that a life-threatening and usually fast growing tumour was pacified.

2008

Six months later I suspected that something was wrong. I asked for a new MRI and discussed my suspicion with Thoresen. He believed that any deterioration possibly was due to him overlooking a weakness in my energy balance, and therefore it could have been a miscalculation on his part not to give me treatments in the last two months. MRI also confirmed my suspicion by showing weak growth in an offshoot of the tumour.

This error fortunately did not aid the development of the disease. After a new treatment by Thoresen the symptoms were less bothersome, and both PET CT and CT then documented the effect in the late winter and spring of 2008. The images showed that the tumour size was back at the level it was a year earlier (according to CT from spring 2007), and those suspicious lymph nodes in the pelvic area were now smaller. My own judgment, which was essentially based on the changes in faecal thickness, was that the tumour had now reduced in volume. Review of various MR gave the impression that the radiologists had concentrated the measurements longitudinally in the intestine. There were no results related to the volume of the tumour in the descriptions.

PET CT showed according to Gustafson an extraordinary "clean", i.e. a metastasis - and mutation free image of the body. The images were cleaner than those normally shown by healthy people, because we all have mutations that lead to the formation of cancer cells different places in the body. This is not dangerous for healthy people where the body itself destroys these tributaries to cancer. The pictures of my body showed only a tendency for such activity in the tumour, but with a value from this technology measurement unit that not with certainty can be said to imply something pathological.

The winter of 2007/2008 was a thriller-like display of how sensitive the immune system, or rather what in our organism that controls cell growth, was to the alternative treatment I got. Without going into detail at this point it should only be mentioned that during the spring it emerged a clear sign that the body itself was now able to control the cancer. The subjective representations on this was that the ME symptoms improved, depression tendencies were completely gone and the stool more normal than in three years. Thoresen had also considered the body's energy balance as stable for four, five months.

The many tissues samples and various forms of X-ray images (MRI, CT and PET CT) was the unbiased, professional medical confirmation that the body had regained control. Although I in all ways experienced and regarded myself as well, the original life-threatening tumour was still present as a foreign element in my digestive system. Nor was I confident that the yet unknown reasons I became sick could not induce the disease to return. Therefore, I still wanted to be followed up by technical controls at the hospital.

In late February 2008, the same day that I learned that PET CT images showed an extraordinary "clean", i.e. a metastasis- and mutation-free image of the body, I was advised by my oncologist Gustafson that I could not keep coming for controls of the disease in the hospital if I still resented to undergo the prescribed hospital treatment. This message surprised me in the sense that it made no sense. While she explained to me the wonderful news of how effective my own immune system against cancer now worked, she communicated a "deal" on a treatment with a new chemical antibody, *Avastin*. This contradiction combined with the shocking possibility of being deprived of the regular controls of the tumour, made me blind to the ethical issues and that this was something I should not decide on at the time, but at least "sleep on it" and maybe also confer with my GP or other qualified advisors. In retrospect, I have been thinking it was just the idea of coming home and talking about this that made me gave in - along with the description that this was a harmless treatment that did not have any of the detrimental side effects of chemotherapy, radiation and surgery could entail. I took the threat seriously and made the decision on the fly. That refusing treatment, which according to the description could also have positive aspects in relation to a final determination of tumour characteristics, was not something I should let lead to a serious conflict in the relationship with the health care system at a high level - something that I much later realised was the unlikely outcome. Today, after being well introduced into medical ethics, I see the threat as "empty". But still very effective at the time it was made.

What Gustafson told me about the treatment was that Avastin had so far only been given to terminal patients in combination with chemotherapy and in order to provide patients with prolonged life. I was offered this antibody without also having to take chemo, as I had earlier refused to take medicine that acts detrimental to the immune system. This was due to my conviction that it was precisely the immune system that was my true healer.

Avastin alone would by description only affect the blood supply to the tumour and thus shrink it. Furthermore Gustafson explained that according to the research on Avastin, any tumour that is really cancer, shrinks considerably. In other words it seemed the only risk being that Avastin would not shrink the tumour so that nothing would happen. This amounted to me as no risk, but rather would be a further confirmation that I no longer carried a cancerous tumour and that the lump in my gut now mainly consisted of connective tissue - insensitive to the Avastin. I had no reason to doubt what Gustafson told me, and I figured it was explained to her by those who were behind this "offer" - probably in collaboration with one of the experts in trials of new cancer drugs at the Radiumhospital's Cancer research department.

In my situation I saw no choice. I thought it impossible to come home and tell that I had lost the chance of future controls in a hospital because I had refused the offer of a completely harmless treatment. I did not realise the absurdity to participate in such a medical experiment, as the first in Norway, probably the first in the world that was not dying and who were given Avastin without chemotherapy, *while all samples and pictures indicated that I was healthy!*

So I accepted the offer and went home and told about the wonderful PET CT images.

The tumour did not shrink. Instead it swelled. In two months it was up in volume that caused a severe impediment to the stool. The result of the new PET CT after completion of the therapy, showed a dramatic increase in activity in the tumour - from 7 to 15 on the scale radiologists use as a yardstick. In other words, the tumour had gone from a size that was slightly below the limit established for pathological activity, to one that was very far above.

The reason that the tumour was allowed to grow for over two months after the photos were taken, are unknown to me. I thought "no news from the hospital is good news" and did not ask for the results of the pictures before my digestion without warning was about to close up. After getting the radiologists conclusion, I went straight from the hospital to Thoresen. I did not tell him what I had just learned, just that I needed a control. This time I was especially concerned about whether he could really read any of what had happened by this almost mystical diagnosis form: taking the pulse at the wrist, not the pulse which provided information about heart the rhythm, but about the energy cycle that acupuncture influences.

He quickly pointed out that the energy balance was now worse than at any previous measurements, including the first time I came for treatment after receiving the cancer diagnosis.

What the hospital soon announced, via MR images, was that the tumour had grown into the surrounding muscle tissue and described it in my medical file as "likely inoperable", which I know oncologists regard as incurable, so they can only offer palliative care.

For the third time Thoresen was able to show the acupuncture treatment's effect on severe cancer. Almost immediately after the needle stick the symptoms improved: In a few days it changed from "rabbit droppings" to a more normal stool.

CT images taken six months later showed that the tumour had shrunk back to the size it was before the Avastin treatment began. All signs of spreading, which I later learned was common "side effects" when Avastin was given without chemotherapy in mice, were gone.

That Avastin has the effect that it had on me, when used without concomitant chemotherapy, has been proven by studies where this has been attempted in mice. Several published studies confirm this. A summary of these is published in the world's largest scientific journal, the American *Science Magazine*. This I learned a few months later after Thoresen on his own initiative had sent inquiries regarding experiences on Avastin into his U.S. network of clinicians.

Research on Avastin given to mice shows that even a few remaining cancer cells, like my tumour were on the PET CT measured to be below the threshold for pathological cell division, for yet unknown reasons may be stimulated both to create new resurgence of the disease and spread to other organs - if no chemotherapy is given concurrently with Avastin. This also explains why it is a medication for dying cancer patients: where it will not be the same disaster if the known side effect affects some of them of their own wish and without pressure of any kind take this opportunity to extend and possibly improve the end of their lives.

11. Chi and Chemistry. A meeting with the molecular biologist Sergio Manzetti

The most important thing is to wonder, ask questions, relentlessly doubt all authority. Constantly try your thoughts against reality.

Dr Lawrence Krauss,
professor of particle physics

Manzetti come by road on a sunny spring morning, to my surprise in one of the smallest and most obsolete car models that will ever come to be parked outside our carport. I knew from before that Manzetti had left a well-paid job, working for the pharmaceutical industry in Australia and had been meeting an uncertain economic future in the face by a far more idealistic motivated work with Thoresen, but still...

The next surprise is the athletic figure that comes out of the condemnable vehicle. Neither in suit and tie or white lab coat, as I half unconscious, half awake, had seen him for me the times he and his research has been featured. He is dressed for summer and casual, with the "right" cut and fabric pants and a tight t-shirt that is abundantly filled with a well proportioned body volume.

The fact that Manzetti has Italian and not Russian bear-genes on the paternal side, was incomprehensible. But genetics is not the theme, and it did not take long after I had these thoughts, that the impressions from the arrival faded and gave way to the introduction to the most compelling research stories that will ever come to be told in our gazebo at the bottom of the garden.

The book of Manzetti´s life and work is not my task, at least not now[34]. Instead of trying to convey his intensity and commitment or relay the many captivating stories, I should write only about the research results he achieved step by step to pursue Thoresen

126

hypothesis, and the steps are long. He takes me on a research trip starting at Blindern in Oslo, continue to Indonesia, India and Malaysia, further half way around the world to the U.S., across the Atlantic to England and finally back to the United States and the first dawning of scientific understanding *why* Thoresen´s treatment is effective, and a further confirmation that shows *how* it works.

The hypothesis is described as one of "bridges" in the chapter of the same name (Chapter 6) and is here summarised as I had noted before meeting with Manzetti, excited to get this in more detail.

The idea came to Thoresen from others acupuncture research. Earlier it has been noted that various documented effects of acupuncture treatment, as pain relief and anaesthesia, are transferable among individuals via blood transfusion. This must be because the treatment causes a formation of active substances in the blood and acupuncture´s mechanism of action can be described scientifically by a biochemical or microbiological approach. By finding and synthesising these substances the effect can be repeated through ingesting these substances in the form of synthetically produced medication. Being able to prove the effect of acupuncture by actually producing a synthetic cancer medicine was for a time also an ambition for a group of patients and colleagues. The main reason that this strategy was abandoned in favour of streamlining the presentation and expanding the trial of acupuncture treatment[35] is described in Chapter 7 ("Meeting with Thoresen").

oOo

It is the 21st of May 2011 and Manzetti has managed to follow the Earth's journey around the Sun thirty-six times.

On the basis of my health I usually experience intense people as gruelling. Manzetti, however, brings a form of intelligent engagement that makes the impact on me the opposite, and it is almost possible to believe him that at the time he was on the lab tour with Thoresen´s blood samples in the Far East in 2006, he did not sleep in four intense exciting months. There was all too many important and exciting things to think about.

The scientific cooperation with Thoresen started in Oslo, Norway in October 2003. There Manzetti made the first and crucial discovery: the premise of being able to initiate a scientific landscaped testing of Thoresen´s hypothesis. He then worked as a research fellow at the Institute of Bioengineering and Thoresen had come by to give him two blood samples. The first was taken just before he did acupuncture on himself, and the other essential blood sample was taken one minute after acupuncture treatment.

Earlier acupuncture research had confirmed the transfer of relief of pain of an animal (A) to another (B) via blood transfusion from A to B, which was explained by the fact that the endorphins formed by acupuncture treatment of A, were still active in B after blood transfusion.

Thoresen postulated that if they found a difference in blood samples before and after acupuncture treatment, the substance or substances that this difference is attributed could have the same effect on someone other than the one that received acupuncture treatment - if the different constitution could be identified and synthesised.

Manzetti found a surprisingly large difference in the concentration of peptides in the two blood samples: equivalent to 1 gram per. litre, which is a huge difference to a molecular biologist, especially considering the short time interval between the samples.

This was six months after Manzetti had first been introduced to the hypothesis. Previously Thoresen has given me the following description of this session:

> - *I gave a lecture in Oslo and finished by describing how it can be possible to translate acupuncture treatment to a chemically manufactured medication. When I finished, there was a large man running through the room, yelling:*
> - *This I can help you with!*

Thoresen recognised him as a young student he had given treatments to a few years earlier, sent to him by his father, Fabio Manzetti, a Norwegian-Italian who had translated one of Thoresen's books into Italian.

At the time Manzetti was Thoresen's patient, he was on his way to his academic life. He had a strong desire to be a scientist and searching for the secrets that hide behind the concept of the placebo effect, known as a generic term for improvement or healing which for unknown reasons is caused by the body itself, often on the basis of strong *faith* - faith that recovery is possible or likely. He had not yet met Thoresen, and he knew nothing about that the latter through his professional life as a therapist and researcher had reached the same ambition: to explore what is in his vocabulary called *self-healing*.

Shortly after Thoresen had solved a serious health problem for Manzetti, the first stone was laid on each side of the bridge, five years later they decided to bridge the gulf that separates eastern and western medicine.

Before the next building block fell into place, Manzetti had completed his studies and gained his professional experience through research in Norway, Switzerland and Australia - research that nearly destroyed his health once more. Immediately it is somewhat difficult to understand that the robust and athletic figure had six episodes with collapsed lung and a heart issues.

Furthermore, he tells about devastating hardships when employed by two of the world's major pharmaceutical industries, but he does not tell why - only that he discounts ever resuming this type of cancer research.

What he emphasises as positive from those years was the cooperation with Ross Barnard, best known for having developed a new technical platform for detection of infectious agents. Manzetti smiles broadly when he says that Barnard liked to refer to them as "the two mad scientists who were surrounded by just normal". Judging from Manzetti's energy level it was easy to imagine that he obviously meant a creative and results-oriented form of madness.

That Manzetti found a difference between the two blood samples at all is the first and crucial step away from acupuncture as magic and superstition. On the contrary, it opens for a research project in which he and possibly other molecular biologists can continue working to identify the changes in the blood that is highly likely to be caused by acupuncture treatment.

Nonetheless, the find turned almost out to be a *nose fish* (expression by fishermen´s conviction that if one of the fishermen get a fish right away and long before the others, there is a danger that he does not get any more - at least not for a long time). Having ascertained that there was a significant difference in the blood samples before and after acupuncture treatment, the next challenge was to find where the difference was. When a molecular biologist talks about *where* in a blood test, it does not mean a "place" in the blood geography, but when I inquired further about this and other things I did not understand, it gave birth to many new questions. However, I found that *where* easiest translates to *what the difference consists of.* Instead of referring the details, I refer particularly interested readers to Manzetti´s own description or the even more detailed disclosures from the U.S. research laboratory that repeated and summarised the previous experiments - both are in this book's appendix.

Manzetti did not find *where* or *what*, but he made an important discovery during the next laboratory experiments in India, Indonesia and Malaysia: he namely found greater complexity in the blood structure in humans than animals (horse), not to mention that it was even greater complexity in blood structure in sick than in healthy people. This is quoted with Manzetti´s explicit prejudice:

> *- These results and other results of my work as you will mention in your book, must be verified by further tests before we can draw definitive conclusions.*

The most spectacular that happened in those laboratories in the Far East where Manzetti purchased research space and services in 2005/2006 was that he had to promise to marry the daughter of the laboratory engineer at a university laboratory in Malaysia. It was the condition for letting him in the laboratory at an affordable price. This engagement could have cost Manzetti considerably more than the money he saved. He had been too focused on the research to think

130

about what kind of religion and law was in force in Malaysia. There it is 'in fact forbidden to associate with unmarried Muslim women without a chaperon, also for foreigners. As he described it, he and his fiancé was alone several times in places where it could have become a basis for prosecution, even if they had not done anything illegal. It's not easy to prove what was not done in this field, when you did not have witnesses.

It had been three years after the nose fish. The satisfaction of having ascertained a difference in the blood samples was reduced to the frustration of not finding out where you should look in the "the wilderness" human blood represents for a molecular biologist. The output that would reveal the qualitative differences in blood samples remained identical. Finally, just before he was about to give up, while he also began to realise that he should get the longest possible distance from the impending marriage, Manzetti got the idea that the difference may be located within the portion of the prints where the graph peaks at the different physical prints came so close together that they could not be separated and therefore visually appeared to be identical, *though they may not be identical in the blood samples*? Maybe the printer was not sensitive enough and the lines too thick?

oOo

I experienced Manzetti´s way of thinking and his attention to the core of the problem as an example of the ideal scientist consciousness - one that is not out to prove or protect anything, but seeks to uncover new, fruitful knowledge. The conditions were many and long, and in keeping with scientific theorist Karl Popper's stringent testing of hypotheses[36]. I am not qualified to judge Manzetti´s general academic qualifications, but I understand through others, not least through the review made by the researchers at the Norwegian Radium Hospital of the laboratory tests, that they are implemented as they should, to be considered by colleagues to be reliable. What I am more qualified to judge, is the man I have in front of me, and the principal aspects of the research that concerns him.

Something that in my eyes reinforces this positive impression and assurance of his accountability, his expressed scepticism about the commercial side of research projects which have medicinal purposes. He returns to the time he worked for the pharmaceutical industry, and the discomfort he still feels to what he later describes as having prostituted himself.

When Manzetti hears of my own reflections on commercial or non-profit objectives behind medical research (referenced later), he makes a surprising comment.

- The pharmaceutical industry is in such a strong financial position of power that no independent research institution, not even national governments, have made the contest and tried to develop cancer medication from a purely medical motivation. My experiences with the pharmaceutical industry makes it impossible for me to wish that they at some point will take over ownership of what I have tried to do with Are. Then they use it to promote their own interests, which preferably is of a financial nature. This means that they will continue on the basis of Are´s and my research, but from an entirely different objective than the one we have.
- *But are you not concerned that your research finally leads to a new medication?*
- Not really. I wanted to help Are documenting his treatment method to those who have the power within health care, and independent research institutes. If I can help to prove that Ares newly developed acupuncture treatment is effective, and that other independent cancer researchers can understand the cause of this effect, I have reached my goal.
- Can we not work for both?
- Only if the scientific research will be continued by independent researchers. Medical research should be funded by public interests which recognises research as an expense, a portion of an expense budget, and not primarily looking at research as an opportunity to make money. It will be much cheaper for society if they can see the cost of drug therapy in

conjunction with reduced costs for medication developed by the community as a whole and not just by a few huge, private industries.

Ares medical thinking and treatment can help the fight against the cancer threat. It is not possible to make money, but it is possible to save huge costs on it. This does not only apply to the industrialised countries' spending on cancer treatment today. Just think of all the productive work that is lost in these countries!

Manzetti emphasises the latter part of his enthusiastic posts by for once to speaking at a leisurely pace and with a touch of authority. And I recognise the depth of what he presents here.

- You probably know the difference between renewable and finite natural resources. An example: Nature creates renewable resources for power companies by lifting water from the ocean and dropping it onto the Norwegian mountains. It is always flowing to the major power reservoirs, and nature will continue to fill them in the foreseeable future.

Have you, who has studied this and seems to be an intelligent person, yet not thought about that cancer diseases creates by far the largest renewable resource for the world's fastest growing industries?

I was taken aback. Silent. I thought: Might this be possible? I thought, no, it couldn't be possible. And thought again: Could it really be possible?

Manzetti had possibly experienced something he could have told us, yet chose not to tell, and I felt that I did not know him well enough to ask. He was finished with the topic and let the issue hang in the air between us while he whispered something that we might address ourselves to the brunch I had talked about. Then I could keep asking about what happened after he escaped from the bride in Malaysia and across the Atlantic to the laboratory at the University of Iowa.

oOo

A solid snack was needed to compensate for the energy that was expended by the large, intense man the first few hours. I had barely consumed half, ate only a third, and before Manzetti picked up the napkin that had blown down on the slate flagstones, and for the last time wiped his mouth, I had a formulation finished. I ask if it is adequate for his views. Maybe I can put it in his mouth in the book - when he has finished chewing:

> - The development of drugs and particularly the question of this research´s direction is a far too important social issue that economic interests should be the parent and the greatest motivation.

He nods and approves the remark. I was again tempted to go a step further and ask him about his personal experiences as a researcher for the pharmaceutical industry. At the same time I thought that he had to choose what he would tell me. Instead, I continued the summary of the surprising perspective he had submitted before we ate.

> - *As you first said, to medicate sick people is a cost. This should not be profitable for some, but a cost the community should carry at all levels. How it works today is increasing profitability for a few owners of medicine production when the cost increases for the rest of society.*
> - Yes, when the most people are sick and patients needing treatment for the longest possible time. The last century cancer patients have increased and they are medicated for a longer time.
> - *But you cannot connect the pharmaceutical industry to the increase in the incidence of cancer?*

- Of course not. I just want to remind the fact that it almost exclusively is researched on cancer drugs that prolong life, not drugs that make patients healthy.

I let the subject lie instead of asking if he had made any reflections as to whether this had been a controlled development and not a coincidence.

- The reason that I went into partnership with Thoresen was that I could use my knowledge to find a scientific explanation for the original "medicine" – the acupuncture method. We have developed more than enough secondary chemical medications. Instead of producing more we should begin to sort out which of them we have that we really need and what we can stop using, i.e. when the ratio of low efficiency and dangerous side effects are a negative calculation. Instead, we can conduct further research on primary healing and especially on traditional strategies that interacts directly with the external nature and our self healing inner nature - that we currently only have a single medical term for.

Manzetti tracked us into his favourite topic, placebo. No matter how much his though to sort and reduce chemical use in modern medicine resonates in my consciousness, this is yet another example of how his energy derails from my original agenda this morning.

- *A while ago you said: "If I can help to prove that the acupuncture treatment is effective", but as I understand it, you have not only helped, but actually proven the acupuncture method's efficiency through the thread of what you discovered in Oslo, and what happened after you left the East and went to the United States.*
- No, no, do not write that. There are too many possible sources of error that must be eliminated through repeated trials, preferably by other and equally independent

researchers like me, and tests must be supplemented by many more that can exclude sources of error and chance. What you can write, is that the responses we have received from our laboratory research, is *an indication* that we are on the right track. You do understand what I mean, I hope - the huge difference within research between indication and proof?

I nodded tentatively, knowing that it was only now, after Manzetti´s many reservations; I realised I still had much to learn about the differences in the legal and scientific requirements of proof and evidence.

oOo

At the end of this chapter, we will follow Manzetti further on his circumnavigation - via Malaysia, on the run from a marriageable Muslim, across the Atlantic and to Iowa, United States. It has become June 2006 and it is now it really is starting to become something that not only researchers, but also people should be interested in.

- I was right. The difference was in the area where the graph peaks in print was so dense that it was possible to hide the differences between the two blood samples.
- *It must have been incredibly exciting to try to figure out what this difference consisted of?*
- You can imagine what I, who are used to seeing atoms, molecules, and proteins as big as houses, felt when a September day at the University of Minnesota...
- You had moved again?

The disruption just slipped out of me. We have now come to the sixth lab, in the fifth country in the continent.

- Forget about that. Sometimes there are even better reasons to choose another university laboratory than a threat of

marriage. University of Minnesota was still an appropriate choice; for it was here that I managed to identify many new peptides, which later proved not to be found among those who had previously been described by other researchers.
- *How many peptides are we talking about?*
- Many. You have to imagine that there already are mapped perhaps fifty thousand different peptides. I chose twelve that had similarities to known protein structures, and can be related to cancer, and took them with me to the University of Massachusetts...

From central (Iowa) to north (Minnesota) in the U.S., and now north on the east coast. Maybe Manzetti had become homesick. He was closer to Norway than ever on his long journey, as close as he could get without starting swimming. But before he started the journey home, he had to undertake the crucial test of whether this work at all had something to it with regards to the overall objective, which was to show through scientific laboratory research that it can not be excluded that Ares acupuncture treatment has effect on cancer.

This would not have been much to write about if it had not succeeded Manzetti to detect such an effect. How it succeeded, really is worth writing about, not least because of the remarkable and rare fact that it succeeded on the first attempt.

The exceptional in this are not obvious, but is specifically for cancer research, which normally attack symptoms from "outside" in the sense that one constructs numerous varieties of substances that constitute foreign body's for the body from a hypothesis one has established regarding the properties and the effect the drug must have in order to have an impact on the disease.

The university laboratory in Massachusetts December 2006, the twelve selected peptides that came "from within", in the sense that the body itself had produced them, placed in test tubes with the kind of highly aggressive breast cancer cells that had plagued the woman who had given the blood samples. Simultaneously, the same breast cancer cells were placed in test tubes with the recognized most effective chemotherapy currently used as medication for this type of

137

breast cancer. The peptides showed efficacy in all trials. According to Manzetti the effect varied between ten and one hundred per cent of the effect of the chemo that were tested in parallel with the peptides. He would not say more beyond emphasizing the usual provisos about several attempts, preferably also with other blood tests and done by other researchers, and so on.

So far in the process the hypothesis is from what I can understand, without detected vulnerabilities, and it *may* therefore be accurate. That the reservation is highlighted is due to the aforementioned difference in evidence in court and in research. For those readers who are not interested in academic correct formulations, but wish and hope for an effective treatment of their cancer, the reservation can be perceived as beating around the bush. They want to know in simple words: Do Manzetti´s research support Thoresen´s hypothesis and does it give any confirmation about the acupuncture method´s efficiency or not? To this question there are at least two answers.

The scientific we know from Manzetti´s many provisos and Karl Popper's philosophy of science.

The personal, that is my point of view, is based on logical conclusions from my own experiences. Further strengthened by the fact that two of the foremost researchers within Manzetti´s disciplines have concluded that there is evidence that the newly discovered peptides have effects on cancer cells in vitro[37]. I think it is difficult, if not impossible, to justify this effect to anything but the acupuncture method, which in nature´s marvellous ways created peptides, which further triggered the reactions in the body which is the more probable cause that the patient was cured. In a logical and mathematical perspective, it appears impossible that this chain of events may be the result of an equally long series of coincidences.

Beyond these initial responses I will to my best ability continue to communicate the facts of the events surrounding Manzetti´s laboratory investigations. The conclusion belongs to the future. Yet some of the future appears already in the following, where we follow Manzetti on his travels after the stay in Massachusetts.

Before I go any further, I will dwell a little more on results from Massachusetts: *Between ten to one hundred per cent of the action of the chemotherapeutic drugs that has cost tens of billions of dollars to develop*, and now sold worldwide as the absolute best medication against the growth of cancer tumours and metastases. Moreover, the chemotherapy 's effect is limited to the time they are in the body[38]. *The naturally formed peptides however, are neurotransmitters that initiate an organic process that lasts.*

Manzetti is not talking about this, as such thoughts do not belong in a scientific article. However, they belong in my opinion in the book. A step further in the chain of thoughts will be to imagine the fundamental difference in the effect this may lead to outside the laboratory – in the human body. If two substances - chemotherapeutic drugs and peptides - basically have as much immediate effect and chemo is rapidly degraded, whereas peptides initiate a latent immunity, we are dealing with two levels of effect: *life-prolonging* and *curative*.

In connection with this reflection I continue with other thoughts I made about Manzetti´s discovery after he left:

• What I know no one else has managed to establish: a natural process in the body that have significant effect on cancer cells, proven by research team Thoresen/Manzetti in the first attempt.

• How would the "world" reacted if one of the major drug manufacturers had announced the discovery of toxic-free substances produced by the body, and as early as in the first laboratory experiments show the same effect on cancer cells that the strongest chemo? And what if this discovery had been given to health authorities in the countries that were willing to investigate further along this track?

I dare myself to make a guess: It would not have been a single health ministry in a democratic country that had not bowed and thanked if the result and privileges of this basic research was given to the community, so that this country's health care system could go in the lead of the eradication of cancer as a deadly public disease.

But - this discovery is made! It has happened in reality, not just a hypothetical example. The only thing that was hypothetical in the example was that it was a pharmaceutical company that had made the discovery, and not two independent Norwegian researchers outside the authorized research communities.

It was the confidence in Thoresen´s medical expertise and the hope to make the discovery that he had predicted, Manzetti had with him in his luggage when he started the world tour. Manzetti found no evidence that the prediction was wrong. However, he found a logically coherent chain of circumstantial evidence pointing toward it one day finally being proved.

oOo

There were no signs that Manzetti thought there was something special about having identified and tested newly discovered peptides that showed effect on cancer cells. He knew of course that what he had found, probably was the next link in the chain events after the needle prick - what made the body of the woman who gave the blood sample capable of itself to stop an attack from a fierce breast cancer. From his professional point of view, the molecular biologist´s, where proteins appear as something at least as realistic as the rest of us experience with our five senses, Manzetti discovered at least a portion of the gun the body even after a millennium long development has found as the best defence against cancer. He betrayed not a hint of professional pride in this or any need for me to portray it as ground-breaking work.

oOo

Sergio Manzetti came home for Christmas and into the next year he went to England, to the University of Nottingham, which has gained wide recognition for its cancer research. There, he began collaboration with a professor who wished to establish a doctoral

140

program in further research with Thoresen´s peptides. This partnership failed. Here Thoresen and Manzetti each has an explanation to why. Instead of referring them I will limit myself to refer something they do agree about in what happened at the University of Nottingham. Namely that their stock of peptides and several of the blood samples that were entrusted university laboratory personnel was destroyed without any satisfactory explanation. According to Thoresen this fact is not easy to explain as an accident.

If oriental medicine was the medical technical basis for Thoresen´s discovery and hypothesis, the scientific seven-mile steps happened in the West. After the debacle in England, Manzetti went back across the Atlantic to the United States and the fourth American university laboratory at the University of Michigan. We have reached May 2008.

Now the animal testing starts. According to Aftenposten (Norwegian national newspaper) with the source of Oslo Cancer Cluster it is required an average of half a billion for laboratory research prior to the commencement of animal experiments. Thoresen and Manzetti came there for a thousandth of this, which they explained by what is mentioned above, namely that when working within and *with* nature, one can go straight on instead of having to look for a "needle in the haystack".

That fall, the peptides were injected into mice that had induced cancer. The first series of experiments showed effects on tumours, averaging 4-5 % growth reduction, which is too small to start human trials. The second essential condition for human trials is that the medication's toxicity must be identified. This was almost a foregone conclusion given that the body itself produces the medication.

A natural progression would now be to follow up these experiments to expand the repertoire of peptide combinations and dosages (quantity and increments). The first series of mouse experiments however, is far the only one. There was no money for more tests. The limited financial resources they had at their disposal, were instead used on a so-called RNA- trials. This is also termed *mechanism attempts* because the goal is to identify the mechanism of the substances for which previous experiments have shown effects on cancer cells.

Before the mechanism attempts Manzetti had as mentioned found indications that the peptides had effects on both breast cancer cells and tumours in mice. If he managed to get on the trail of the mechanism, it would narrow the probability that the good results of the other experiments could be due to anything other than the peptides, as impurities in the samples, which he himself said, among his many provisos.

Early experiments had shown as mentioned a "disarming" of cancer cells. Manzetti succeeded through the RNA attempt to show *how* the peptides disarmed them. If anyone has so far harboured doubts that the peptides actually have an effect, it would by showing how they work, by logical necessity remove any justification for such doubt.

The RNA attempt showed that acupuncture treatment, just one minute after the needle prick had changed the genetic basis of the patient. Such changes are called epigenetics.

Epigenetic factors are believed to be important in tumour development and also in the development of the organism, and probably also are of importance for evolution in general because the genetic repertoire increases.

Epigenetics is defined by Richard C. Francis in the book *Epigenetics*: "The term epigenetics is often defined as changes in the genetic material that does not include the DNA code, but which nevertheless changes the function of genes. Typical examples include methylation of the DNA molecule and the acetylation of histones which DNA is coiled around"[39].

Then there were initiated preclinical trials (trials with mice). However, these attempts had less effect than the in vitro experiments. That the peptides at all affect tumours in living beings is regardless a breakthrough. Another important factor is that these trials whatsoever did not show any toxic effects on normal body cells.

As an amateur in scientific research, but with a certain proficiency in literature, I once more take the freedom to formulate my own summary of Thoresen and Manzetti´s findings, based on both their statements. I am in fact not concerned with test tubes and petri dishes and weeks and months of repeated trials, identical or with slight variations, to arrive at the truth. I see a straight arrow - except for the frequent movements back and forth between continents. This journey did not set out to prove anything or to map *the full truth*, but to show scientists and laymen, healthy and sick, that the bridge between Eastern and Western science can be developed through the approach from both sides now conducted by Thoresen from the east and Manzetti from the west.

In case of a positive result of the recent laboratory experiments Manzetti performed at the research laboratory at the University of Michigan in 2008, he would have completed the entire series of experiments with the exception of improved animal and human trials. The following were then obtained:

- evidence that acupuncture causes large amounts of new substances in the blood
- identification of new substances
- documentation of the effect on cancer cells in laboratory test tubes
- documentation of limited effect on cancer cells in mice and no toxic effect on healthy cells
- documentation of the mechanism

Manzetti says that also the mechanism attempts succeeded in the first series of laboratory experiments. What he found is that the peptides control - *regulates the level* – of the genes, as previously shown, is involved in aggressive breast cancer. Thus it is no longer just the series of Thoresen´s patients that confirms the efficacy of treatment, but a complete series of laboratory experiments, where no one form the so-called weak link in the chain.

What any attempts with industrially produced copies of the peptides in cancer patients will demonstrate, is if the acupuncture treatment´s positive effect can be copied in the same way as it is done for other synthetically produced peptides.

Through my work on the book, I have the understanding that medical research is an extraordinarily laborious process. It must be when it costs in the order of billion dollars to develop each new cancer medication[40]. Although if Thoresen's hypothesis is correct and Manzetti´s laboratory trials are error-free, there are processes that remain, which are the most costly. If the purpose is to develop a new drug, these challenges are met by handing over primary responsibility and control to a commercially motivated player. As the situation is today, the few transnational companies that decide which cancer drugs are to be developed and marketed have a complete monopoly, as they each develop their various drugs, and because they are the only ones who have sufficient financial resources for this work. They each have their patents, a "scheme" which further reinforces the players' positions and secures it perfectly camouflaged cartel. That it has become like this, is because of the American system, where the lack of public healthcare necessarily entrusted private medication production, and how the patent system is the way they defend their investments in a corporate jungle battle for profits. In Europe, however, the nation's health care system could have collaborated to produce medication, without regard to outperform each other. In such a partnership will "the others" success become everyone's benefit.

As it has become, I imagine that it is the democratic countries where human rights are strongest and thus the care of residents' health - such as in Scandinavia - that conditions are best to compete with those who have profit as the main motivation. In particular, Norway itself, with the backing of an oil fund, which can easily reallocate the funds so that we can investigate the curative medication and treatment methods without fear of that the market shrinks along with the tumours. Then the health budget will shrink accordingly.

What fascinated me the most and was left hanging in the foliage long after Manzetti had gotten his once white car to start, was the combination of intensity and truthfulness. I imagined various analogisms born of the collaboration between the muscular gunpowder and the sometimes extremely relaxed Thoresen, with his ability based on nature's little hints to draw deep and far-reaching conclusions. This is a property research colleagues may see as superficiality, but constitutes the condition for Thoresen´s main fields: the combination of an intuitive and rational endowment to uncover nature's own ability to heal itself.

The rust spots on Manzetti´s car when it was fleeting between the foliage and let out one last salute from the horn was for me the hallmark, both symbols and evidence of an atomic- and molecular-artist who has followed his strong desire to be independent and no longer work towards the goal he did not see any qualitative value in.

oOo

A few days later, while I rounded off the work to shape this chapter, Manzetti called and asked if I had heard about the price increase on Algeta shares on the Oslo Stock Exchange. I had no idea what Algeta was and thought Manzetti was the last that followed the stock exchange. It turned quickly out that it was not there he had heard about it, but in the mainstream media news of June 6th 2011.

While he is telling me about this, it dawned on me that Algeta is the source of one of the many good news about an upcoming cancer drug on the market in recent years, which was first in the media in the time just before I started working on the book. At that time there was an agreement with drug giant Bayer who had sent the stock price through the roof.

Two days after the news of Algeta was released and Manzetti had called me about this, the financial news on TV2 reported that the share price was now thirty times higher than it was two years ago. This time the accelerating financial adventure was due to information about the trial of Algeta´s medication Alpharadin, and that it showed approximately 7% extended life of prostate cancer patients with spreading. This meant an expected overall increase in prostate cancer market in the same range, namely about 7% since the prostate cancer survivors would then consume on average 7% more medication. It was precisely this the news was about, and it was turned up like a giant novelty, which it also was within the financial world. But if it was received as giant news by the patients with prostate cancer, which in a couple of years when Alpharadin is released on the market can hope for a mean extended life of 3 weeks is questionable.

On the other hand, this week's major stock exchange news is undoubtedly bad news for the western countries' public finances, which will cover the cost of the medication. It is not a question of small amounts. The company calculates the three weeks' longer life to cost the health care system 35,000 dollars pr. cancer patient. The market that Algeta/Bayer covers, consist of the approximately 100,000 men under hospital treatment which each year die of prostate cancer. Assuming that doctors believe the three extra weeks' life is worth 35,000 dollars, the new medication will annually cost society more than 20 billions NoK.

Algeta´s share of the calculated profit is estimated at 15 billion NoK total in that time they have patent protection. I would think the big player in the partnership, Bayer, is getting a much bigger profit. All these billions is the price that is calculated by Algeta and Bayer, and which they can calculate in advance because they are protected by the monopoly that arises partly because the medication is patented by the private and non-public market.

So far I have described a treatment method that in an easy and affordable way could cure a significant proportion of the 100,000 prostate cancer patients. Certainly, the laboratory research presented in this chapter is made on the basis of aggressive breast cancer, but in clinical practice, the acupuncture method proved to mobilize a defence against most cancers.

So far in my work I had only interpreted the Norwegian academic community's strong opposition to Thoresen as a result of personal competition and prestige factors. After the conversation with Manzetti I had a new and far more dramatic situation to relate

146

to: the industry that currently produces the cancer drugs, is fully aware that if anyone - whoever it might be - is launching a life-saving cancer drug, all other cancer drugs, which substantively prolong life, become redundant and manufacturers lose their livelihoods.

12. Anecdotal healing and natural cancer treatment

I detected no cases of cancer, so if there was any, it must have been very rare.

Albert Schweitzer about the health-state of Gabon in 1913

As one of the few who had passed the heyday before I experienced cancer in my immediate family or circle of friends, I had not gained any more knowledge in this field than one would naturally through the media. I had reached a point in my occasional surveys about cancer diseases where it no longer was enough with general considerations and philosophical reflections. Especially when it came to one of the fields that affected this book's main theme - the background to the consistently strong contradictions between authorised and alternative viewpoints - I realised that my general knowledge was not enough.

My own starting point has been what I also believe is the prevailing notion, namely that cancer is a deadly disease, but that in my lifetime, well over half a century, there has so far been major improvements in the understanding and treatment of the disease, and that there are also a few alternative views that seem to have some substance. This is especially what I see as the core of *natural medicine* - what consist of what we consume and what it contains of plus and minus factors in this context.

As soon as I wrote this, I pondered over that the question of what we take into the organism, is emerging as an alternative viewpoint to the authorised cancer research. That foodstuffs, and for that matter lifestyle, is not a central element in authorised cancer treatment, is becoming more and more strange the more I read from qualified research in this area. It is not only authorised and alternative

148

medicine that acts as rivals, but the same inconvenient competition also takes place between two branches of natural science: food research and research related to combating the symptoms.

The next and really big surprise I got is that there has not been as much progress in the treatment of cancer diseases as I initially thought, especially if you compare it with what has been achieved in combating other deadly diseases. This surprise together with the topic I brought up in full in chapter 9 ("About the laboratory research") - the so-called *anecdotal healings* - led me to the first real aha-experience I had since I started on this work, that it almost without exceptions are researched on what goes wrong in the body when cancer develops, instead of how a healthy body combats disease in its first stages. This resulted in the chapter "The mystery and the solution", which the following sections are cut from:

> "It has in fact never been researched on other patients than those receiving the treatment that always has been considered the most effective and which consists of different forms of removal of symptoms - either by surgery, chemotherapy, radiation or various combinations of these methods. For ethical reasons, it has not been possible to recommend patients to take the risk by retaining symptoms through a research project. This has prevented scientists gaining knowledge about what happens in cancer cells, tumours they form and the body in general in patients where the growth of tumours are either inhibited, halted, or where tumours become smaller and may completely disappear through self- healing."

A possible consequence that there is no research on cancer cases where the disease has declined by itself, is that such a development has been considered to be extremely rare (anecdotal), yes also inexplicable and almost unnatural. Hence the unscientific collective term cancer researchers and doctors have given this form of healing.

149

The more I thought about it, the stranger this phenomenon became. I decided that authorised cancer researchers *must* exist who have been curious about how such natural healing occurs. Something else I regard as almost unnatural and incompatible with "research nature". And I decided that with the same necessity something *must* have prevented them from communicating what their curiosity led to of new discoveries or hypotheses.

Finally I found a German scientist, Lothar Hirnreise, which for years has accumulated knowledge about the so-called anecdotal healings. He is half-way within authorised medicine through his medical training and practice, and half off because he found his research material mainly through the study of alternative therapies.

Through Hirnreise´s research, I finally got a well-documented confirmation of my hunch that healings that occur outside hospital cancer wards, are either particularly rare or unnatural. My conclusion was then that the most inexplicable healings had remained unexplained for very long if it had been a goal to give them a scientific explanation like Hirnreise works toward.

Through the readings of Hirnreise combined with my newly acquired knowledge that cancer research for generations have constituted the basis of existence for the commercialised industry, it began to form an answer to the question of why this has not been a goal. I would think Hirnreise himself would have formulated the answer like the following:

> - It's just a question of what who pays for the research wants you to find or research: chemicals that prolong progression of cancer or natural defence strategies against getting sick or stopping the disease.

oOo

Prior to this sad conclusion led to a final determination on my own viewpoint, increasingly squeezed as I was between alternative and authorised medicine, I read an article about a Norwegian cancer researcher who had a strong focus directed at precisely the fact that nature itself may be the best, and perhaps the only real healer of cancer.

Unlike the notion of natural healing as very rare exceptions, a view which so far has been a dogma within authorised cancer research, cancer researcher Jan Mæhlen, Professor of Pathology, Ullevål University Hospital, has in Dagbladet´s Magazine (Norwegian newspaper magazine) 27.02.2010 given the public a very different picture of cancer diseases than what you get when you focus primarily on late-stage disease, i.e. when it has reached a stage which in most cases leads to a fatal outcome:

> *Analyses indicate that two of the three tumours detected by X-ray, would have disappeared by itself.*

I had now got a surprising confirmation from a renowned cancer researcher that the recent cancer research is starting to get on track of *what is right in the body* (cf. chapter 3 ["The riddle and the solution"] and the above quote), what constituted the basis for Thoresen´s search for the solution of the cancer riddle thirty years ago, and what his treatment is based upon.

This statement led me to contacting Mæhlen half a year later to make sure that Dagbladet had quoted him correctly. When I referenced to the notion I thought was the universal, namely the opposite view of the Mæhlen expresses, he replied that this is not based on research but only on assumptions and beliefs, as I had already indicated in my text (above). There is no older research on this. On the contrary, any new research indicates that cancer come and go, and generally *without being detected.*

In other words, the so-called anecdotal healings is the most frequently occurring outcome of a cancer disease.

Naturally it is "something" that causes the healing, but this "something" is thus processes in our organism which *in the quiet -* quietly and unnoticed until young cancer researchers have recently become aware of it - overcomes the disease.

Before this date, I had only heard one researcher unequivocally state that a majority of the tumours disappeared by self-healing. Mæhlen confirmed that this view represents a generation shift in cancer research. It is not a matter of just a change of the former view, because if these new research results are widely recognised, this will almost overnight lead to a domino effect in that a number of "pieces" falls within both research and treatment that today relies on the dogma that cancer diseases are irreversible.

I could tell Mæhlen I assumed that I also in my younger years had been suffering from colon cancer and that the disease had withdrawn with no other reason than that I quit smoking[41]. That I came to this conclusion, although my former primary care doctor dismissed this as a sort of phobia of cancer, was due to a realisation that at the time appeared to be obvious: I never understood that physicians and especially those dealing with cancer statistics, had not seen what I saw, namely that there was not an explosive increase in the number of cancer cases, but that improved methods of diagnosis together with a rising public fear caused smaller tumours inevitably discovered long before they reached a stage of disease with a greater right could be described as irreversible.

When cancer statistics began, there was no offer of diagnosis until the disease had evolved into an advanced stage. For some reason it was therefore assumed that the dogma of the population are as many early as advanced cancers - which also would have meant that the cancer diseases are irreversible. As improved diagnostic methods revealed tumours at an increasingly earlier stage of the disease, long before tumours became noticeable, so that treatment can be started earlier, one should have observed a similar decline in the diagnosis and treatment of advanced cancer - if the disease is irreversible. The statistics from the mid-nineteenth century onwards, where the improvements in diagnostics was the greatest, shows no corresponding reduction of advanced cancer that should have happened simultaneously or in parallel with the large increase in the number of early treated did not happen. The only logical explanation for this relationship is *that the number of early developed cancer cases in the population are much higher than those that develop through to advanced cancer, that for a significant number of the early treated the disease would have retreated again - without treatment,* as Jan Mæhlen confirms is now discovered through his and others' research.

That a number of *smaller* tumours shrink back and disappear with no known cause can still be described as anecdotal healings in that medical science does not yet know why *the number of early developed cancer cases is much higher in the population than advanced cancer,* but because it no longer fits well within this term, I would suggest that *self-healing* or *natural healing* is more aptly. That this is so, and the fact that scientific research (according to Mæhlen), Are Thoresen (which with this as a starting point has achieved extraordinary clinical results) and I have reached by different routes - should in my view inspire authorised cancer research to prioritise this field of research.

Mæhlen´s presentation of recent research results give us two new alternatives to the dogma that cancer is an irreversible disease.

• Either nature's own self- healing is about as effective as hospital treatment, or
• Self-healing is the major cause of all healing, even where the patient is undergoing hospital treatment[42].

By this it is natural to conclude that it is the missing knowledge about cancer´s "natural course" - that is, when it is unaffected by treatment - which has helped to maintain the general notion that it is solely authorised hospital treatment and nothing else that can alter the disease´s inexorable path towards death. This is such a scary notion that so far only four of Thoresen´s hundreds of cancer patients through thirty years who have dared to rely on the immediate improvement his treatment has given and not as a "precaution" also undergone hospital treatment.

As I immediately see this, cancer clinicians throughout the modern medical history has taken all the credit for something just as much or perhaps entirely is the work of nature, meaning that no cancer is cured without the help of self-healing or somehow is stimulated to contribute. This would not have been particularly worrisome if it had not been for a serious "side effect" associated with such notions. This side effect hits with full force the groups of cancer patients whose treatment has not had the desired effect. They are told that because the treatment does not work, they will come to die, a message, which in itself can be fatal. The psychological impact on the course of the disease is basic knowledge for doctors who are not only familiar with placebo´s curative effect, but also with its counterpart, negative beliefs or *nocebo*[43], and what kind of health problems this mental condition can cause. An often-used example of nocebo is the story, true or false, about the man bitten by a harmless snake, but confused it with a species he knew was deadly, and died.

For cancer patients, both the diagnosis and subsequent notion related to future suffering and death may be a factor as devastating as the physical symptoms. It's no easy task to turn the nocebo effect that has been set due to several generations' prejudices about cancer.

Mæhlen´s references to recent research on the dynamics of cancer - their growth and withdrawal - is a crucial first step towards exploring strategies to help nature or the body to eliminate the disease itself. One result may be that nocebo will be replaced by placebo. This presents both opportunities and responsibilities, not least by the changes we can make in our lives to help an overwhelmed immune system to recapture its original strength.

To form a reasonably well-founded picture of alternative views on cancer and directions in cancer therapy did not seem insurmountable, not least thanks to the amateur researcher's favourite tool: the Internet. To penetrate deeper into what cancer research and cancer treatment has been and is, appeared on the other hand as an almost hopeless task for someone who does not have a medical degree.

However, there is a shortcut to a overview - statistics. Through my own experiences and a new review of the patient diary I became aware of several surprising facts that rules the sometimes-cryptic know-how and research terminology, which probably could ultimately mislead the public. I followed this path further by checking

154

the Cancer Registry's web site, where a very extensive statistical material is presented. Some surveys were especially adapted patients and those with general interest, and they went as far back as even I could remember (over fifty years). In this connection, I tried to get a professional substantiated picture of what form of treatment of the three main forms - surgery, chemotherapy and radiation - was the most effective.

The unexpected answers I got through my simple studies of the statistics, including that at no time it was possible to find some improvement in the statistics that could be related to the development of new treatments or drugs, lead me to seek professional help to find out if I had read and/or interpreted the statistics wrong.

My statistical surveys were not a goal in itself. What I wanted was the most truthful understanding and comparison of different forms of cancer treatment represented by the main categories *authorised* and *alternative* therapies. With the exception of vitamin D[44], none of the different treatments or lifestyle advices I examined, were even close to the results Thoresen obtained with his method.

It was not just some of the public statistics that gave me major negative surprises. Parallel to my work on the statistics I decided to carefully examine the form of alternative treatment that for me has long seemed the most promising, namely the so-called vitamin B17, synthesis of a bitter substance extracted from apricot kernels. Here I found a serious defect in the given references, which *may* indicate fraud.

Faced with little trustworthy information on both sides of the chasm between the alternative and the authorised treatments the work on the last part of the book took a slightly different direction than planned. Instead of limiting myself to consider natural cancer treatment based on the available information, and rely on it, I had to provide a credible comprehensive picture as possible of *truthful* information. It was much more difficult than I had imagined, especially because so much of the information had few and more or less worthless references, and because it was difficult, and in many cases, impossible to verify them.

To the best of my ability, I had to thoroughly search the sources to identify the facts and avoid unsubstantiated claims or obvious forgeries, which expanded the scope of the book considerably. The few persuasive strategies I found within alternative therapies had the same position within the treatment hierarchy as Thoresen´s treatment method: surprisingly good news, but probably with a long and winding road toward use of their full potential. Along with a *possible* significant effect of certain vegetable triglycerides, i.e. vegetable oils with high content of polyunsaturated fatty acids, these natural treatments led me to a third category of treatment, which I place between the authorised and the alternative forms of treatment, and as I have described as *natural cancer treatment*.

By this I do not mean that existing alternative treatments are not based on helping our natural immune system to overcome the disease. This I believe applies to the majority of them. The reason for introducing this term is that it hopefully can moderate the contradictions and bring attention to the fact that natural processes are superior to the unnatural and that it is against the disclosure of nature's own defences against cancer one should put the research resources into.

Mostly thanks to the knowledge of Mæhlen and his colleagues, MD. Per-Henrik Zahl, a senior statistician at the Norwegian Institute of Public Health, research natural cancer treatment now appears in my eyes as a full-fledged science-based alternative. Their research involves a completely new understanding of cancer as a disease in which the *potentially dangerous* symptoms in approximately two-thirds of the cases retards completely independent of the treatment. I write "potentially dangerous" because it is only to the extent that abnormal cells or tumours not retarding before they damage other tissues or organs, cancer symptoms are a real danger to our health or welfare.

For me this was perceived as having discovered a goldmine with virtually limitless possibilities.

At one time, natural healing of cancer was portrayed as almost a metaphysical phenomenon and given, in a scientific perspective, the

156

derogatory term anecdotal healings. Now is the time to turn this around and realise that we actually have an effective defence against cancer and that this supremely is about physiological processes that are no longer metaphysical or mysterious.

Seen in a larger perspective where acupuncture meets science, Thoresen´s treatment method is no more mystical or metaphysical than that the right impulse from the acupuncture treatment may lead to the formation of new peptides that may function as neurotransmitters. Such signal substances are common in the body. For example, white blood cells produce interleukins (signalling proteins) as part of the immunological defence mechanisms.

Through this biological cooperation, as of yet is far from fully explored, the "life energy" - *Chi* (China), *Prana* (India) and *vitality* (European medical designation) – ensures our *life force* (European folk-term) and health.

What pushed me so strongly to tackle this project was the first glimpse Manzetti and Thoresen gave me into our own biological marvel: that we ourselves are in possession of a natural cancer medication.

Basically, I will not deny that knowledge of a natural cancer treatment in general has made me sceptical of alternative treatments that do not arise from the organism's self-healing powers. The alternative methods I knew from before, and that does not directly support the immune system, but involves proper nutrition, detoxification and stress relief - strategies that can be very significant, but not strictly a treatment method - is not something I personally would have selected. With the knowledge I have today, I would neither have selected a method that adversely affect the organism's self-healing before I had tried if Thoresen´s acupuncture method could stimulate it. This may happen in parallel with the surveys that is always taken between diagnosis and treatment in a hospital can be initiated. Time will not be lost if Thoresen´s treatment does not have a measurable (biopsy, MRI) effect and one may then initiate hospital treatment instead.

I opted not to go deeply into the study of alternative treatment methods, when I by various investigations have found no convincing evidence that there is a method that provides greater power than nature itself can - with the exception of treatments related to nutrition and lifestyle, which I found even more interesting and believable. Nutrition and lifestyle is indeed supremely about nature and what it basically manages itself, but as we in some contexts deliberately have to magnify to achieve the desired effect.

Something I've always meant and thought to find within alternative medicine is a more faithful management of important parts of our heritage, which authorised medicine has pushed into the background in favour of modern chemical drugs. In the former, I see opportunities to develop future cures in the same way as Thoresen has found a base for his treatment method for cancer within the acupuncture technique.

When I gaze up from the way it is, and to what it may be, the question arises as to why alternative medicine really stands outside the health care system. Seen with fresh eyes, it appears almost unnatural for a highly developed society that the public health system only engages actively in a limited part of the total health care system.

It's not only I who has realised this. A first step towards a *comprehensive* health care system was the establishment of the organisation NAFKAM (National Research Center in Complementary and Alternative Medicine [www.nafkam.no]) under the University of Tromsø. This work will hopefully open the door for the health authorities taking the alternative into the heat and deposits a mite of their financial and technical resources to develop a form of cooperation that also can provide so-called alternative researchers better opportunity to document their activities. This can be done by *qualitative studies*, which I in the next chapter will show may be a cheap alternative to the hugely expensive quantitative studies only major pharmaceutical companies have the financial means to carry out, and that helps to maintain the sharp distinction between authorised and alternative (*naturally*) medicine.

oOo

With regards to diet and lifestyle that strongest have been shown to affect cancer, is what we are getting directly from our physical existence's primal source - the sun. Similarly, photosynthesis in the plant kingdom, the premise for an overgrown planet, the sunlight is forming the life-giving properties of our blood that we so far know as the instrumental designation vitamin D. The research on the medical effects of sunlight led in the Norwegian side of the aforementioned Professor Johan Moan, professor of physics at the University of Oslo and head of the department of radiation biology at the Norwegian Radium Hospital. With his group of researchers, he is a key participant in an impressive international research network[45]. By reading up on this research's "destiny" and the impact it has *not* had, I realised in earnest how difficult it is to direct research towards simple, natural and affordable solutions when it comes to the cancer problem.

The two known external factors influencing the incidence of cancer in a global perspective are climate and lifestyle. In 2007 The National Hospital published a summary of studies that were adjusted for other variables – cultural factors, diet, lifestyle etc. – that in this type of study could influence the results in a way that can make them more or less worthless. This summary showed a declining cancer incidence at lower latitudes. On NRK radio Moan said a year later that statistical calculations show that the optimisation of the climate factor (natural vitamin D by sun exposure of the skin) of the Norwegian population will reduce the number of deaths due to cancer by as much as 10 cases daily. Over a decade, this corresponds to the entire population of a medium-sized Norwegian city. If this is the case, this knowledge will virtually overnight revolutionise the cancer problem.

The second external factor that provides significant variations in incidence and cure of cancer, the culture and lifestyle factor, is easiest to analyse through what we eat and drink. There has been research in this field for more than 100 years, and those who in recent times have coordinated this research have been able to deal with almost 10,000

159

studies[46]. Virtually all of these studies conclude that one or more examined foodstuffs are particularly favourable or unfavourable in terms of preventing and in some cases to reverse the development of cancer. My immediate thoughts that our hospitals adds little to no weight on these factors[47], is due to the notion of cancer as an irreversible disease that only authorised cancer treatment can stop or hinder - that is, through more or less brutal removal or destruction of disease symptoms - and that other strategies have minimal impact on disease progression and absolutely no bearing on the outcome of it.

Nutritional and lifestyle issues are numerous and extensive. I will briefly refer a single study of one of the many so-called supplements (minerals, vitamins, trace elements, antioxidants and others), which concludes with a significant preventive and/or curative effect on cancer. This is in return the most comprehensive and potentially revolutionary study among the 10,000 surveys. The study applies to synthetically manufactured vitamin D (the sunshine-vitamin). In addition to vegetable omega-3 fatty acids (from linseed/flax) is vitamin D the two supplements I through my limited research has come across to have the greatest effect. Thoresen and Manzetti's laboratory research also shows that a side effect of the acupuncture treatment in patients with breast cancer is that it acts regulating on the blood levels of fats, including cholesterol. This effect neither Manzetti nor Thoresen put any specific meaning to until I told them about the revolutionary research that has been conducted on the sunshine-vitamin.

The first comprehensive study of the association between vitamin D content in blood and cancer was conducted at Creighton University in Nebraska, USA. 1,179 healthy, post-menstrual women in Nebraska, USA, participated in an experiment that lasted four years. The women were divided into three groups.

One group received calcium (1400-1500 mg / day), the other received the same dose of calcium plus 1100 IU vitamin D3, while the last group received placebo. In the group treated with calcium/vitamin D the incidence of cancer was reduced by 60 % (sic!). When the study was adjusted for previously undiagnosed

160

cancer[48], the result was a real improvement in breast cancer incidence by 77 % (sic!).

The study was published in June 2007. It was referenced in Aftenposten shortly after[49] and positively commented on by both the Radium Hospital through Moan and NCS Deputy Ole Alexander Opdalshei. NRK P2 has since followed it up with reports of the research program "Good to know" (later renamed "Echo"). Later, however, the revolutionary impact of the climate, sun and vitamin medication against cancer has fallen out of the media's focus and remained a kind of medical secret. Vitamin D *have not yet - five years after the cancer inhibitory effect were scientifically proven* - become a recommended supplement to the traditional cancer treatment.

Someone - with a huge "medical" power - apparently believes that we Norwegians still in an unknown number of years, should miss the preventive effect of natural, free (in the summer season) or reasonable (in the winter: solarium, charter flights) sun-vitamin that would have prevented possibly as many as 70 % of the cancers that continuously affects our population.

Why?

One of the indications of inertia in the absorption of important new knowledge is myself: When I started working on this book project, two and a half years after the publication of the Nebraska study, I knew nothing about this. I thought then that all forms of UV irradiation of the skin were dangerous. What I still however believed, or believed to have a diffuse understanding of was that the development of new chemical cancer medication had improved the situation considerably for cancer patients, a perception I think I shared with the majority of the population.

By pre-calculating the effect of the *natural cancer treatment* we can get by optimising the blood content of the "sunshine vitamin", research has shown the following:

> • Daily administration of 1100 IU (*international units*) of
> vitamin D has in large-scale trials shown reduction of the
> incidence of cancer in American women over age 55 with at

least 60 % (77% by statistical correction for women who entered the study with a non-diagnosed cancer).
• Statistical calculations, prepared by Moans international research network, the optimum supply of natural vitamin D through exposure of the skin by tanning (*not burning!*) could reduce the number of deaths by cancer in Norway by approximately 3,000 or 30 % annually.
• Statistical calculations, published in Aftenposten's A-Magazine 17.04.2009[50], showing that chemotherapy has a positive effect on the chance of survival for five years - which does not mean final survival of the disease. The improvement in life after five years is not greater than 2.1% in Australia and 2.3% in the U.S. No significant curative effect was detected in the largest study ever conducted of the impact of chemotherapy.

Vitamin D and chemotherapy is in other words, two different dimensions of cancer treatment. In addition, we also have the preventive effect of vitamin D, which Johan Moan has informed about in scientific papers and in the media. If we add the statistical pre-calculations for prevention (77 % - Creighton, adjusted for those who already had cancer at the time of the start of the study) and the healing effect (30% of the remaining 23% - referenced by the Norwegian Radium Hospital from the international research network's overall report) we will with a simple calculation arrive at that optimal use of vitamin D in prevention and treatment *will reduce the number of deaths by cancer in Norway by approximately 85%.* These figures show a relevant comparison with vitamin C's effect on scurvy, a subject that is illuminated from a different point of view on the next two pages. Here we observe that cancer is in fact closer to being a "deficiency disease" that can be prevented, rather than a virtually incurable disease that only in some cases can be cured by severe attacks of the disease symptoms.

That our health ministry prefers to support the costly, invasive and virtually ineffective treatment with chemotherapy rather than the cheap, and in its most effective form *the comfortable treatment from the sun*, it is absurd for a layman like me.

What is almost as remarkable in my eyes is that it's not all about unsubstantiated claims from alternative researchers "outside" the public environment, but proven facts in accordance with the best tradition of Science. These facts are obtained by researchers where many of them, not just Moan, is among the most highly valued and recognised in cancer research in the Western world.

Despite thorough research, I have yet to find any reasonable or sensible answer to why, six years after the revolutionary news about vitamin D′s effect on cancer was discovered, it is still radiotherapy, chemotherapy and other costly chemicals that applies. All the while a veil of forgetfulness and silence has settled on vitamin D and effectively prevented what I thought would be managed in a way that would give the world's cancer patients and those who believe themselves hereditary predisposed a positive hope for their own future.

When I shared the results of my research and my frustration with one of those who through thirty years has educated a generation of bioengineers at the university college of Østfold, Elisabeth Astrup, she showed me an example from a textbook in pedagogy which in principle is about translating new important knowledge into useful practice. The example is the first double-blind trial in history. It is from the beginning of the days of sail-ships where another vitamin deficiency disease, scurvy, destroyed large parts of the crews of ships that sailed the clear waters, was long in the sea at a time and therefore had limited access to fresh vegetables and fruits.

I quote from the book *Innføring i innovasjonsarbeid (Introduction to innovation)* by Kjell Skogen and Mari-Anne Sørlie[51]:

> "In 1601 the English ship captain, James Lancaster, led an
> effort within the British navy to cure scurvy with lemon
> juice (vitamin C). Out of four ships it was only the crew on
> one that got lemon juice. Halfway on the journey to India
> 110 of the 278 crewmembers on the other three ships had

died. On the lemon juice ship all were alive and most of them still healthy.

This trial was followed by another 148 years later – with similar compelling results. 48 years after this again, in 1795, the British navy took in use lemon juice as a medicine against scurvy, which immediately eradicated scurvy in the Navy's fleet. 70 years later, in 1865, the British Merchant Navy also took this method in use and the disease was then "quickly defeated in the other European fleets as well..

I am left sitting with the feeling that a form of treatment that would be an adventure and almost getting to paradise - extended winter vacation in a Southern hot country - could almost be called "outrageous" and a way too simplistic and improbable solution for those who for generations have worked out from the ingrained notions of cancer being unresponsive to anything other than authorised cancer treatment.

This could be part of the explanation, but far from an answer to my big question: why nothing has happened from our health authorities in the six years that have passed since the discovery. I had some important gaps in my knowledge that I needed to try filling. A long day of searching on the web followed and a new day of conversations with people I had found out knew much about the history between the discovery and today. This was information that approached an answer, albeit fragmented and incomplete. I will therefore go somewhat back in time and refer what I know now about this matter.

Shortly after the Nebraska study was published, a campaign started against the survey at several websites in the United States. The strongest performer was The American Cancer Society, an organisation similar to the Cancer Society in Norway, but with the important difference that it receives most of its funding through donations from cancer medication manufacturers. This was answered from more natural medicine oriented websites, who pointed out this

164

financial connection. They explain this strategy by that drug manufacturers were already underway to develop a medication based on vitamin D. Until such medication was developed and patented there will be much effort to prevent un-patented vitamin D and vitamin D supplements in foods – while a recovering population will reduce the need for other cancer drugs significantly.

We're used to "that´s how it is in the U.S.". Nevertheless, a few years later the same thing happened in Norway. The Cancer Society´s website and other more official publications from the Norwegian health care system went from unreserved support to the independent vitamin D research and praise of its results to quoting the "counter-research"[52] and creating uncertainty and insecurity associated with increased use of vitamin D by the end of 2010. This is evolving exactly as natural medicine oriented websites in the U.S. predicted would come: *in Norway there is now far greater documentation requirements for vitamin D effects before it can be recommended for cancer patients, than it ever has been raised to new, costly and very toxic drugs before they have been used on Norwegian patients.*

Is it true? I ask again. Is vitamin D suddenly become an alternative competitor to the supranational medical monopoly? A supplement, which overnight has transformed itself from a healthy and absolutely necessary vitamin, is alleged now to be dangerous in doses that a number of comprehensive studies in the wake of the Nebraska study emphatically proved preventive and healing against cancer! Although it is now in accordance with scientific rules of evidence is proved that vitamin D has an unmatched ability to prevent and cure cancer, we are still not recommended to eat more of it or bask more in the sun or no longer drink cod liver oil, so that we certainly in the winter could have achieved a vitamin D levels in the blood equivalent to what our health authorities until now have considered harmless?

Is this really true?

Yes, according to Moan this is unfortunately true. He is audibly upset on the phone while he talks about the "counter-research" and of other radiation researchers which still focus only on the dangers of skin cancer, which is caused by repeated sunburns and not normal tanning. He says that it is now focused on a maximum intake of vitamin D from reasoning that large doses are dangerous, rather than to increase this limit significantly. Moan refers to research that shows that populations who work outdoors or live in climates leading to the highest vitamin D blood levels in the world, up to fifty times what is now said to constitute a health hazard. It is a documented fact that the populations with the greatest so called overdose are the healthiest, not only regarding cancer but also a variety of other diseases in which high doses of vitamin D have proven effective.

I ask if anyone has tried to shake his position as one of the country's most renowned cancer researchers throughout a long career. I imagine that Moan scoffs at the other end of the phone while he says that he has published everything he writes on the topic in the most reputable medical journals internationally, but that in Norway the Medical Journal rejected the resume he wrote in Norwegian to orient Norwegian doctors on the revolutionary new and important topic he detected. He has no explanation as to why, and when I gently ask if he has thought about the huge economic impact this research may have on the pharmaceutical industry and the academic consequences it may have for many of his colleagues, it is clear that he is not familiar with these perspectives. However, I believe it gave him something to think about.

Moan asks me to convey that he welcomes all who are qualified to judge the stack of studies in his office and compare them with the attempts to thwart the facts.

Is it eventually proved that there is something to the conspiracy theory?

For the first time in my life I began to have an interest for this aspect of the matter: the world as conspiracy theorists see it. I had sometimes encountered such in my quest for knowledge, but it was only when I came across an incredible prediction from the time after the Creighton study on vitamin D were published that I found something that aroused interest. I write incredible and can add "but true" because the first part has long since come true, almost exactly as was predicted already almost six years ago in the United States. The part of the prediction that is still future tells us that the authorities will come to halt adding vitamin D in food, as it is today, for example in milk and various milk products, stating that it may cause unsafe and dangerous high dosage, and that vitamin D supplements hereafter be given in the form of specially approved supplements or medication, for example to cancer and MS patients. This assumes of course that the industry succeeded to patent such products. That they will succeed in documenting its efficacy, we know from all the independent studies Moan has referenced. Meanwhile *the conspiracy theory* (which I am now tempted to shorten to "the Theory") claims that the information about vitamin D will be limited as much as possible - something I have described above as the "veil of forgetfulness and silence". Seemingly consistent with this tactic advised intake of vitamin D in the form of sunbathing and solarium particularly with regard to the risk of skin cancer instead of being given factual information about how much sun exposure is healthy as opposed to excessive sun exposure that increases the risk of skin cancer.

According to Moan is the risk of skin cancer present only for people with particularly sensitive skin or excessive sun exposure that causes sunburn. Reliable studies show that occupations that naturally exposed to the sun, such as fishermen and farmers, are less prone to skin cancer than indoor occupations. In other words, *right/normal sun exposure also protects against skin cancer*.

It would have been great if the Norwegian health authorities could confirm that this is just a conspiracy theory, and make sure the Norwegian population optimised vitamin D intake in accordance with the new facts that exist about what is recommended - *regardless of what health authorities in the United States have chosen to do*.

Perhaps we should have a completely independent health policy within this topic and definitely parting with perhaps the most corrupt and patient hostile section within the Western health care system.

This should be an obvious path as one of our foremost cancer researchers who have reached the highest international recognition has presented rock solid research (Moans review) showing that within a decade we could save the lives of a number of people equivalent to the citizens in a medium-sized Norwegian city. Society as a whole will save colossal costs of hospitalisation, radiation, surgeries, expensive medications, sick leave and disability benefits.

After the first conversation with Moan I understood that he has gone from being one of the nation's leading cancer researchers through several decades to becoming the "bad guy" in a medical soap opera he has no idea who is directing. In the international vitamin D research he still occupies the same position he had previously, while he in the scientific community in Norway is close to suffering the same fate as Thoresen: to be silenced to death.

I am left feeling empty after the conversation, with a strange feeling that a whole sector of our society is manipulated, and I probably will never be able to name the manipulator.

oOo

A few days later I dare to make a phone call to another researcher, namely the aforementioned Mæhlen. I then get a new confirmation that we are not alone in our views. This call is for me an even bigger positive surprise than the conversation with Moan, especially because Mæhlen so unambiguously confirms what he has written about cancer as a dynamic, reversible disease, which in two thirds of those cases where it has formed tumours, yet can be overcome by the body's own healing strategies.

Mæhlen has previously been employed at the Cancer Registry with statistics as his field of work, and he immediately shared my conclusions regarding how cancer statistics are used to create a wrong impression of a generally increasing number of survivors. Both issues are central to chapter 14 ("Statistics as a witness").

Mæhlen´s research has long been focused on the effect of the mammography offer now given to all women above 50 years (screening of the breasts to detect cancer tumours). Although this research is not directly related to the topic of natural cancer treatment, it is through this work I became aware that Mæhlen and other young cancer researchers shares Thoresen and my own view of cancer as a reversible disease corresponding to most diseases.

Before I called Mæhlen, I had looked into the debate whether the mammography offer to all are really good or not. At the other end of the phone, I got a committed and competent description of cancer dynamics, exactly as Thoresen had expressed it. Immediately I also had such an understanding of the cancer diseases, but before I became familiar with the mammography discussion, I counted it as impossible to hear such views from a cancer researcher at a Norwegian hospital.

The most pleasing is that he confirmed that there are more scientists out there, who, in their youth, independent of heart, eagerly are looking to resolve issues that have previously been taken for granted without any scientific justification[53].

When mammography was offered to all, the expectation was that an early diagnosis would result in a significant decrease in the number of serious cancers. Had there not been such an expectation, it would have been pointless putting substantial resources to such an effort.

In over a decade, it has been a great deal of disagreement about if the expectations of mammography have been met. Statements from the National Institute of Public Health suggests one, while the Cancer Registry's website claims the opposite. Generally the debate leaves the impression that it is doubtful whether the measure will reduce the number of deaths. If this main impression is correct and the number of serious cases of breast cancer is not reduced by increased use of mammography, it may have several causes.

The most obvious reason, which is also pointed out by cancer researchers that do not support the mammography initiative is the recognition that many of the cancers detected at a relatively early stage, would have gone away by themselves if they had not been diagnosed. In other words mammography leads to too many being treated with the negative consequences this entails. Here I mention only the very first and the very last: the message that you have breast cancer - and that this mental strain along with the other negative consequences of treatment overall leads to a number of women without mammograms would never have noticed the tumour ends up dying of breast cancer. The core of the discussion is whether this last group is larger than the number of women that with mammography detects and get successfully treated a tumour they would otherwise have died from.

This may sound like a matter of statistics. However, one should never forget that it's about real people, and that one can never know who ends up in one or the other category. New knowledge and technologies has put doctors to one of the modern medicine's greatest dilemmas.

I have no qualifications to decide whether the mammography offer should be maintained or not. What has aroused my attention, is a relationship there can be no disagreement around, namely that a high number of smaller tumours that are now diagnosed after the mammography scheme came into force, *has not been shown as growing tumours in older statistics*. Assuming a fairly stable incidence of breast cancer tumours, this is irrefutable, statistical evidence that a similar number of tumours previously disappeared by natural means. Had they not done so, they would necessarily have developed into serious cancer diseases and caused the number of registered cases of cancers before the mammography offer to be radically higher.

Yet another evidence of cancer's dynamic nature.

In short, the professional scepticism to an extended mammography is justified in the professional recognition that treating cancer in certain groups, in this case, early diagnosis of breast cancer, may lead to the opposite of what you want to achieve, and that it was almost taken

170

for granted could be achieved. That it was so, was due to at least one hundred years, perhaps as far back as cancer has been categorised and named, that cancer was considered an irreversible disease[54].

Maybe the intense debate about mammography result in that we get a more "relaxed" and natural relationship to cancer, and thus increased confidence that we can do something about it.

My hope is that this will not be such a long process that thousands of Norwegians will have to suffer and die because those now in power, are clutching to what they learned about the disease when they were young, which Mæhlen was afraid would be the most probable continuation. But, as he said, " the old is the eldest and will first reach retirement age. Then, the next generation of scientists leads the way".

Because it is the "young" research that allows for the understanding of why Thoresen´s cancer treatment have such effect, it's no wonder that I choose to round this issue by quoting from two studies published in the spring of 2012, confirming Mæhlen and Zahl´s study. They are referenced on the website Dagens Medisin (Today's Medicine) and in VG the 3rd of April and is the result of a collaboration between the National Hospital and Harvard University. One of those behind the study, Professor Michael Bretthauer (the National Hospital), was initially a supporter of mammography. To VG he says, however, that the results of the study were shocking and led to him changing his position. Thirty times as many women have been harmed [by unnecessary cancer treatment - my note] as those who have had benefit of the mammography screening, stresses the lead author of the study, physician and researcher Mette Kalager.

oOo

During a brief review of the previously mentioned German researcher Hirnreise´s work I return to the diffuse phenomena *spontaneous* or *anecdotal healings*, and notes that they are far more numerous than most thought[55], both because there is no known medical research in this field and because only a minority of those who experience this, go to the media with his miracle story or contribute in some other way that it becomes known. This may again be because physicians tend to explain away or making this form of healing negligible. The main reason for this collective denial, I believe is due to that spontaneous healing without cause in authorised treatment violates the ingrained notion that cancer leads to death if symptoms are not removed or completely destroyed by the hospital treatment. Given that cancer research has not achieved any breakthrough reflected in an actual defeat of the disease in spite of the enormous efforts throughout the modern medical history of science, the need to protect research reputation has been correspondingly large. This is a possible explanation for several generations of professional obstruction of any notion that there may be other methods or strategies that can prevent and fight cancer diseases. A change in these grim images of cancer may hopefully eventually bring a curbing to the diagnosis destructive effects (nocebo).

A probable surprisingly high number of anecdotal healings did, however, makes it even more difficult for me to understand that they form a complete blind spot within the authorised cancer research. A significant contribution to that I came to the conclusion that the number of anecdotal healing is much higher than most have assumed, is because I was aware of the existence of research on anecdotal healings. Admittedly, a researcher who does not work within authorised medicine has done this. However, his method should interest anyone with a touch of medical curiosity.

Hirnreise has a professional background as a nurse and as a psychotherapist. He did start medical studies as well (without examination due to an early commercial career). He started his research after a friend got cancer and asked him for help to orient himself in the marginal mapped landscape of different therapies. Hirnreise had already sold his business, was well off and had plenty of time. For several years he interviewed all the terminal patients he succeeded in tracing who had survived the death sentence from cancer hospitals by seeking other forms of treatment. Then he examined all the forms of therapy he in this way came in contact with.

172

This led him on many journeys, where he came into contact with many different cultures and treatment methods.

On the background of the gradually more than six hundred interviews with people who were healthy through alternative therapies, he established a list with descriptions of more than a hundred different cancer therapies from all over the world. The material he has collected is collected in two voluminous books. A summary of the contents and his conclusions are easily accessible through search online. These can be a first stepping-stone for cancer researchers and other interested parties who wish to acquire a broader view on cancer treatment.

A specialised research on the items Hirnreise has identified, could be a reliable book and a basic curriculum in the future oncology study. It can not possibly be considered advantageous that the majority of oncologists and cancer researchers remain ignorant about what the different culture- and medical historical forms of therapy against cancer is all about, their scientific basis, and what results can be expected from them. That there are indications that such therapies have the highest number of healings where hospitals have the least makes such an approach and bridge building to something close to a necessity. The book will of course also be welcomed by cancer patients, who would usually only have internet or various alternative therapists to turn to if they do not give up the fight.

What Hirnreise demonstrate as common to almost all these roads towards healing is that they strengthen the human capacity for self- healing. Furthermore, they directly or indirectly, based on what humans alone or with various elements (forces, substances) in our natural surroundings can provide.

A first concrete result of Hirnreise´s work is the establishment of a clinic in Stuttgart, based on the therapies he has seen to make the greatest impact. The therapy I especially want to mention is a diet designed by Johanna Budwig (1908-2003, German biochemist), who among other discovered omega-3 fatty acids major health significance already in the middle of the last century, which was "rediscovered" by other researchers a few decades later. By studying her works, we get a slightly different picture of the importance of the advanced and specialised fatty acids marketed as herbal remedies and medication today. Budwig noted namely that we are best served by ingesting the basic and vital omega-3 fatty acid from plants (flax, hemp and others), because the body itself in most cases converts this fatty acid to one or more complicated variants of fatty acids *if we need it (them)* so we do not risk buying an expensive product that is not what the body has the most use for.

Budwig was several times nominated for the Nobel Prize in chemistry and is thus safely housed within traditional scientific research. Because of her initiatives to radical changes in cancer treatment in German hospitals she met much resistance. As authorised medicine, not at the time or subsequently, placed great emphasis on the connection between nutrition and cancer or nutrients' effects on the course of the disease, Budwig´s cancer research neither then nor later came into consideration.

It is easy to see Budwig´s research as a dangerous challenge to the medical monopoly. Essential fatty acids (i.e. fatty acids vital to the body that it can not itself create) is not patentable and will not be able to be incorporated into some expensive medication. If they are as effective as Budwig´s protocols and results from the clinic in Stuttgart suggests, her diet based on a combination of the aforementioned fatty acids and milk proteins[56] remove a significant portion of the market for cancer drugs, namely the patients.

Budwig´s findings are particularly interesting in the context with the Radium Hospitals research around the fat-soluble vitamin D and Manzetti/Thoresen´s observations of the cancer treatment´s (acupuncture) regulatory effect on the blood´s fat-content. Currently Manzetti only measured amounts of fats, but Budwig´s research makes it applicable also to measure the differences in the balance between the different triglycerides (fatty acids) and cholesterol (fat: HDL and LDL cholesterol).

The most interesting for cancer patients is the importance of Budwig´s nutritional advice from the 1950s is proven to have for terminal patients - including those who now seek the clinic in Stuttgart in the very last hope of saving their life. Put simply the clinical records, summarised in a study of 68 patients recently

174

completed, shows a survival rate of 25%. Corresponding figures for this group of patients in public hospitals is zero or at best a hundredth of a thousandth.

It is also one of the examples that led me to no longer considering the anecdotal healings as miraculous or so rare that they have no scientific interest. I shall not vouch for the numbers from the clinic in Stuttgart. Nevertheless, I challenge the Radium Hospital through Moan, who probably has knowledge of Budwig's work, to convey to the Norwegian population whether her research is in accordance with his own and many others about vitamin D. If it is true that one can both prevent and cure a high number of cancer cases by a moderate change of the diet, which probably can further be enhanced by optimising the vitamin D content of the blood, the Norwegian population should be made aware of it as soon as possible and from the highest possible authorised sources.

Almost as a curiosity it can be mentioned that Budwig smeared coma patients with a mixture of linseed oil and milk proteins, which her laboratory experiments had shown has an ideal chemical structure to penetrate the cell walls and bring life-giving energy to the cells. She placed the beds out under the open sky and fresh air to heighten the effect. Given that it was described that this was a practice that she conducted over a long time, it is credible, though not proven, that a significant number woke from dormancy.

The organisation Cancer Control Society also has much information on the internet regarding different therapies mainly based on natural and healing therapies. Whether or not the information conveyed is reliable or not, I leave to the individual reader to judge, in consultation with a specialist.

oOo

A new Norwegian concept, "cancarian" arises out of an ambition to activate cancer patients according to their own situation and to take responsibility for it. For the cancarian it may not only contribute to a better life compared to being a completely passive patient, as most are today. In some cases, involvement and participation, the experience that their own initiatives have an impact on the outcome of the disease results in that the era with cancer may be perceived as better than the life one had before the disease was discovered. Regarding this I am a reference myself, and I formed subsequently a slogan: *Living with cancer rather than dying of cancer.*

The research director at the University of Stavanger, Olav Helge Bergesen, who launched the concept on the radio a rainy October day in 2010, also confirms that life can become better. This surprising experience I think is because we move attention away from being sick and instead concentrate on what can make us healthy. This can become a self-reinforcing strategy due to a shift in attention and may lead to the discovery of causality that one may suspect has led to the disease, which can put one on the track of things you can do or not do to reduce the pathogenic and depressing elements of everyday life.

The starting point for this new and slightly more upright term *the cancer patient* is a book by David Servan-Schreiber, Anticancer: A New Way of Life (2008). It was released in Norwegian the autumn of 2010 (*Kreft & "terrenget ditt": Hva kan du selv gjøre*, Oslo, Arneberg) with foreword by Bernt Rognlien, a media exposed doctor who is also an acupuncturist. Rognlien is the leader of the Balder clinic, which has as a main purpose to promote natural treatment. This explains largely Rognlien´s major involvement in efforts to facilitate cancer patients' attention to lifestyle and environment, and his emphasis on the possibilities for the patients themselves to improve their life situation and prognosis of the disease. Servan-Schreiber, Bergesen and Rognlien has been joined in this way of thinking by Andreas Olav Stenvoll, head of the Norwegian Oncological Association, which provides good perspectives for future work to improve the overall offer for Norwegian cancer patients.

Bergesen had been diagnosed with terminal cancer a year earlier and had made several measures with regard to his lifestyle that he experienced gave him a better life than he had before he was diagnosed. As the nation's first cancarian he had become convinced that his own intervention in the situation - to "*grab life and change factors one has power over*", as he put it - would also be of great importance for the end of his life.

Regarding the diagnosis and the death sentence, he had full confidence in the doctors. He spoke clearly as he knew he would die of the disease. This absolute certainty that the doctors were right in their assessment, astonished the interviewer, which had to ask again and got the same instant answer.

This answer puzzled and disturbed me so much that I immediately decided to call attention to the fatalism of the prevailing (mis)understanding of what cancer is, has evoked in the entire population. The reason for my unease is that these death sentences, which are distributed more than thirty times a day at Norwegian hospitals, and which a clearly intelligent Bergesen had already received, gave the fatal conclusion that because healthcare can no longer offer the patient any treatment, he or she will inevitably die of the disease. This is a common fixture in the authorised cancer treatment with dire consequences: for example, there is no effective control of over-treatment of terminal patients so that they are actually dying of a health degrading treatment and not the disease itself.

I wrote this because during my work on this book I have passively witnessed the dying process to one of my best friend's mother. His name is Erlend Botolfsen. He has no objections confirming my description of the ending of his mother's long agony. Long before I obtained more information on this issue, I was initiated into my friend's battle to prevent what he described as the murder of his mother because of the over-medication after the doctors had given her the death sentence. He had his reasoned belief that his mother could still become healthy, a belief the doctors did not share. They continued with a treatment Erlend experienced as highly disruptive of life. He told me continuously about this turn of events as it unfolded, and asked me for advice until he finally "stole" his mother from the hospital and took responsibility for her life's ending.

That it went as it did, is something he blames himself for, because he too late ended the discussion with the doctors and took matters into their his hands. His assessment is that although cancer was the underlying disease, the medication was the actual cause of death while it prevented the mother, with his help, to make use of different treatment while there was still time.

I might add that when I first heard about the disease of Erlend's mother, Erlend had no objections to authorised treatment. However, he was sceptical that acupuncture could have anything but soothing effect. This meant that he initially did not follow my advice to seek Thoresen. Erlend changed his view after becoming familiar with the script for this book, which thus first occurred at a time when the mother's body was so destroyed by medications that although the development of cancer shortly after he sought the help of Thoresen had stopped, which is recorded by the hospital´s MRI images, her life stood not to save. After Erlend's assessment it was therefore the failure of other body functions than those who were threatened by the tumour, which led to the death of his mother. The cancer was only indirectly the cause, so that in his opinion it should have been "cancer treatment" as the cause of death on the death certificate.

I could add that one of my neighbours, who lost his wife some time later, had the exact same opinion as Botolfsen. He told his story one day we met in the street, without any knowledge about my book project. When he, after my recommendation, a few days later took his wife to Thoresen, parts of her body, bones and vital organs such as digestion, were destroyed by chemo and radiation treatment, which in this case was fully acknowledged by her doctors. Treatment by Thoresen was also approved by the hospital, but she died of the aforementioned internal damage before MRI images were taken to verify the effect of the first acupuncture treatment.

If it is as I am convinced about: that will, hope and faith are effective contribution to successful cancer treatment the established practice of giving death sentences because the treatment has failed, is to my knowledge of the placebo and the opposite nocebo, for the vast majority contributing to that the death sentence is followed by death. In addition to the nocebo effect causes this advance ruling that the terminal cancer patients lose their courage and willingness to seek second healing strategies. The judgment stimulates human innate

178

tendency to fatalism and means that only some of the patients and their relatives, as Erlend, will be doing something other than focusing on relief of any pain and preparations for the meeting with "certain death".

My assessment of the seriousness of distributing such death sentences is supported by both Hirnreise´s surveys and interviews, and a similar poll recently conducted by a Danish clinic that accepts terminal patients. A larger number of patients who have survived this change in strategy - for example, to seek such a clinic instead of passively waiting for death - has in this study answered which single factor they believe has had the greatest impact on their survival:

- decreased intake of harmful/toxic substances
- increased consumption of health -strengthening substances
- strengthening of internal, psychological factors

Both Hirnreise´s and the Danish clinic study shows a large majority in favour of internal, psychological factors.

If Hirnreise´s forays into the white spot on the map as the anecdotal healings represent, are accepted as the valuable pioneering work it has actually been, the spreading of expertise in this field can help to unsettle the described and little fertile ideas about cancer diseases that have hindered exploration, development and progress of natural, effective treatment.

oOo

The questionable in this situation is not only the one-sided emphasis on economic merit of those who produce the chemical drugs. In addition, it has meant that we have forgotten - or at least discarded - something essential in our own recent medical tradition, as we know through the still vivid images of the wise and ever-present house-doctor.

This loss was pointed out by the head of NAFKAM, Vinjar Fønnebø, in a radio interview in connection with an international conference held in Tromsø in the summer of 2010. Furthermore Fønnebø was concerned about if the human medical factor, as Thoresen more specifically refers to as the importance of the intention from the clinician, can be an overlooked element in the trial of some forms of alternative medicine. Removing the homeopaths from the study of homeopathic medicine and allows the preparation alone be the subject of investigation, we remove such an essential part of this treatment that this is a likely explanation for why this type of studies show worse effect than the homeopaths clinical results from a real treatment situation. Nor is it certain that either placebo or the preparation is the effective in this form of treatment. It may be interesting combinations where *both* factors are important for the treatment to be effective, and we know next to nothing about it, simply because they have never been investigated.

In my reflections on these matters, I have taken a step further and asked the question whether or not the intention behind the production of the drug also has implications for how the drug affects the patient's health.

In a historical perspective it is a relatively new phenomenon that it is not primarily medical professional motives behind the development and manufacturing of medications. The obvious question then becomes whether there may have been some fundamental impact on medication's effect that the main intention behind their development and production today is shifted from wanting to help others with their health problems to earn the most money possible for the producers?

I guess that for many readers the hypothesis about the motivation behind the drugs as an active element in the treatment be very little consistent with the basic notions of the existence of a physical reality that is insensitive to mental processes, that it will be dismissed as pure fantasy.

To this I ask if it has not always been so when a new conception of reality is about to replace some of the old: the traditional beliefs have to be changed so that they are consistent with the new findings? As we know, this happened when Copernicus' mathematical calculations showed that the sun and not the earth was the center of our solar system. At that time science had to change several basic notions in their cosmology.

There is however no new discovery that mental processes influence physical processes, and Fønnebø may, in light of new published studies rely on the discovery that mental processes have identifiable physical characteristics. These physical characteristics have the property that they affect related, mental and psychological processes within other people. Thus overcoming the barrier of physical distance as regards to the dissemination of mental processes between different creatures, such as feelings, emotions and the will to act.

These newly discovered nerve cells are termed as *mirror neurons*. These have got their name because they trigger an event in an individual by mirroring another individual movements, i.e. they are active at observed activity performed by others[57].

If Thoresen, Fønnebø and the mirrors neuron researchers' assumptions about the importance of intention of the clinician or doctor has some truth to it, they notions that are associated with the most dangerous diseases, especially cancer, potentially be a serious, perhaps the most serious aspect of the disease. Cancer often progresses very rapidly after the patient has been diagnosed, although it may be many years from cancer cells beginning to form a tumour to the disease being detected, may be an indication that the diagnosis has become a serious part of the disease rather than a first step towards healing, and that it has given the cancer better growing conditions in that the resistance is further weakened.

oOo

Modern medicine has sought to develop drugs that work most predictably on the largest possible population independent from the wise house-doctor. This may be a general feature of our cultural development, namely that *inner* qualities and skills deteriorate in line with the development of *external* aids. As such, the explosive increase in chemically derived drugs has taken over for the GPs development within the subject and the relationship with the patients.

Modern medicine has largely succeeded in its ambition. However, the success has been mixed, not least because most GPs now know the chemical medication´s side effects. Another factor is whether the medications make patients healthy, or if it is more about local and temporary symptom relief, and that in reality there are very different conditions in the patient's life and environment that determines whether he or she is healed or not. Or there may be other forms of healing methods, which primarily sought after basic conditions that are the root cause for the occurrence of serious disease symptoms. To find and change these deeper causes is the intention behind both acupuncture and several other forms of healing that has achieved great historical and geographical distribution. Unfortunately, they are still perceived by our health care system largely as competitors, something I do not to the same extent as previously thought to be based on real medical professional grounds. After becoming aware of the close links between industry and modern medicine, I think this connection is the true cause of this contest, and that the patients are the real losers. The competition takes place between colleagues who all have as a subject and profession to alleviate disease and therefore have everything to gain by cooperating. Seen in a "bigger" perspective it seems that superior "powers" are organising a kind of academic cockfight between professional athletes that should have embraced each other and mutually appreciated each other's professional resources.

A Serbian surgeon who has for many years worked at Norwegian hospitals, Milan Spasojević, told me that a big part of medication use in Serbian hospitals after the war(s) that followed President Tito's death and the dissolution of Yugoslavia was replaced by acupuncture treatment. This was mostly for economic reasons, but to his knowledge it had no negative impact on the hospital´s treatment results.

In Norway, there are still two conflicting views among physicians about if acupuncture treatment has an effect beyond placebo, but in recent years there has been a positive development in terms of increasing the use of acupuncture in hospitals. According to a new survey published by NIFAB (National Information Center for

Alternative Therapies, an institution under NAFKAM) acupuncture is used today (2013) by every fourth Norwegian hospital.

I would point to a project at the Hospital in Vestfold (SIV) where breast cancer patients are offered acupuncture treatment to soften the sometimes serious side effects of the anti-oestrogen therapy most of these patients receive. The treatment is based on studies conducted at Henry Ford Hospital in Detroit and presented at European Breast Cancer Conference in Berlin, April 2008[58], and in a smaller study conducted at the Hospital in Vestfold by Jill Hervik and Odd Mjåland, surgeon at Sørlandet Hospital (the South Coast Hospital), Kristiansand[59].

In the news at the time of this writing, the focus is on a particularly low incidence of cancer in Eskimos.

Low incidence of cancer with people living in synch with nature is a so obvious and evident phenomenon that it would have been detected and attributed great importance long ago if the research had only seen in that direction. This phenomenon, I believe was first described by Albert Schweitzer (1875-1965) in a report on the state of health in Gabon (Africa) in 1913:

> *I detected no cases of cancer, so if there was any, it must have been very rare.*

On the way back through the history of culture we encounter an issue that is so obvious and so significant that it is strange it has not been thoroughly investigated:

Why is not so that the societies and cultures that have not made extensive use of our treatments, affected by cancer to a much greater extent than is the case?

There should have been a greater incidence of cancer of the so-called primitive societies than in the civilised. At least if cancer research consensus is correct, namely that cancer is not significantly affected by diet and lifestyle, and that it is an irreversible disease that only

Western, technological medicine can heal. I have arrived at three possible answers to the question above:

> • Either because people in so-called primitive societies live in ways and in settings where cancer does not occur to the same extent as in the communities that have undergone Western medical treatment, or
> • because they are cured by anecdotal healing (self healing) or alternative therapies or by the wise tribal doctor without any hospital treatment or
> • because they are healthier because they are neither diagnosed nor treated by technological/chemical cancer treatment

It is possible that the cause is a combination of two or all three answers. There is no deeper research behind them. Especially the last answer cancer doctors will probably dismiss as an outrageous question. Yet this, in my eyes, is the most interesting option. There are two reasons for this:

Firstly, because especially young cancer researchers, who do not share the traditional view of cancer as a deadly disease, believes that the *over-diagnosis*, for example through the offer of mammography screening to all, may increase the number of breast cancer deaths since one then also run the risk of over-treating, i.e. treat cancers that otherwise would have regressed by itself (by self-healing).

Secondly, because this is easy to check. Access to extensive statistical material on the web makes it easy to judge our technologically advanced cancer treatment´s efficacy compared to the large number of patients that new research has calculated has been healed "by itself", i.e. without any conscious intervention by modern technology. We will return to this survey in the next chapter.

Part IV

Status quo or a peaceful revolution?

13. Is it presented evidence for Thoresen´s treatment method?

I must confess that the statistics for me has been a superficial but nonetheless interesting acquaintance until I began to examine cancer statistics. During the reading of my own notes in the patient diary quoted in Chapter 9 ("About the laboratory research"), I got an eye-opener in terms of how a closely related field, *probability calculation*, which sometimes uses statistics, other times just abstract mathematics, can be used in our context. What I describe as *pure probability calculation* in contrast to *statistical probability calculation* (statistical significance) is not based on a large number of trials, but in a qualitative study of individual cases. This method is used scientifically to strengthen claims or test hypotheses that there is basically no statistical evidence for - simply because the topic is too narrow or that for various reasons are not in the focus of research or public interests involving the keeping of statistics.

It may be advantageous to refer back to Chapter 9, page xx, where there is a more complete description of the two main forms of scientific research and evidence.

Generally speaking science go boldly into the new and unknown, not to mention being open to trying other research methods than oneself are trained to use. This noted with a satirical look at the testing of new drugs, where the only approved method for approval of a new drug requires hundreds of volunteers to determine the statistical probability that the product has proven efficacy.

The road from the *statistical* probability calculation (quantitative) to pure or *general* (qualitative) probability calculation is as mentioned not unknown in scientific research. In other areas of medical research than testing of medication, and in most other branches of scientific research, it is established satisfactory probability by a few qualitative experiments, in some cases, just as few as "the only one" without lacking establishment of statistical significance and in any way making these research results questionable. Anyone may ascertain this by browsing some of the so-called popular science magazines or follow equivalent TV shows or at best by consulting publications in scientific journals. The overall picture shows that pure probability calculation dominates as documentation method, and that it is rather rare to see statistical significance used as evidence or proof of a hypothesis[60].

A crucial prerequisite for a single experiment may be accepted as satisfactory evidence or proof, is that it excludes any human or technological disturbing factors. The example in the note below represents one extreme of evidence in scientific research in that it completely lacks the quantitative element - it is solely about a single example/test. The method used in drug trials, represents the other extreme in that all qualitative elements is omitted. It is free of subjective judgment or other forms of qualitative assessment, but is based on pure counting of individual results.

The qualitative method focuses on the specific results of the survey, a result that depends on many different factors and details that might occur during the experiment. The description of these factors, such as extraordinary experiences participants may have had during the experiment, is often part of the final evaluation of the results.

The other and quantitative method focuses solely on the answer to the main question posed in advance of the experiment, usually just a yes- or no question - such as: Does the assayed preparation have positive effect on the disease or not? The result is determined after counting, trusting that the mathematicians are right when claiming that a large enough number of participants statistically will come to correct for possible sources of error (human error, equipment failure, etc.) and randomness (as in our case it is what the so-called anecdotal healings are considered to be). Everything that happens in the course of the experiment, and that does not provide a certain statistical effect - at least one in a hundred in drug trials[61] - are weeded out in the final result. In this way only what is related to the main question is cultivated: How statistically likely is it that "this or that" is the case, for example, if a drug is effective, have side effects or is downright dangerous?

When I wrote the story of the imaginary researcher mentioned in the book's third part, I had on two occasions been treated with Thoresen method with positive results. I did not know then, that there would be a third time, which would become the most immediate and convincing healing of them all.

Meanwhile, I had on a trip to the other side of the globe and at large enough distance from established notions of what research methods should be used and in what cases, discovered that my illness was a type of single event that principle had adequate research relevance - even if it so far was "only" two examples of effective regression of cancer.

This discovery I saw as so interesting to assume as a starting point that I took another step and made a simple statement of my case's premises and results. Though it is done amateurishly, it is hopefully not less illustrative for readers at different levels of interest and professionalism. To secure me against my own amateurishness leading me astray, I asked Nils Hjort, professor of mathematics at the University of Oslo with statistics as research area, to read through this and the next chapter, where statistics are a key issue. Although this was neither statistics nor mathematics at a high level, it was a reassurance to establish that there was no failure of reasoning.

It appears that both doctors, medical researchers and particularly those who manage healthcare investments, have blindly accepted that half of the tools we have at our disposal to assess the drugs benefit or harm, is scrapped. In my view, the most important half is rejected, namely the tool that not only relies on a quantitative analysis, but mainly evaluates a drug or treatment methods qualities. What I have in this chapter's introduction has described as the *quality* of qualitative research, will hopefully make it clear that it should be any investigation and discovery's first basic step, the industrial pharmaceutical research has omitted. I ask myself how it could have come to this: *Who* has decided - and *why* – that those who decides which drugs we are offered, accept that society can take on an average of ten billion crowns on a mainly secondary quantitative study[62] of a new drug effects, such that it can be approved or not for use in health care, while it is ruled out that a cancer medication may be developed through a cheap and predominantly qualitative study?

oOo

There are usually two stages of proof. The first concerns evidence in relation to the present case, which is being examined. It is described here as "qualitative proof". The next step concerns evidence that this single case has transfer value to identical or similar cases, that it is evident that it concerns other patients with rectal cancer.

The first part of "our qualitative study"[63] consists of the following components:

> • A serious cancer diagnosis: malignant tumour of 3-5 cm near the rectum (difference in observations and photos), operable under question, which requires prior radiotherapy. Statistically overwhelmingly likely spread to the liver, lungs etc., and very poor statistical prognosis for survival.
> • The day after the diagnosis a half-hour trial is carried out with Thoresen´s acupuncture treatment at a cost of four hundred and fifty NoK.
> • Based on the hospital's investigation the following month: two series of CT and MRI images to assess growth and various tissue samples, determined that the tumor is not growing anymore, and that it is only found cancer cells that "is no longer cancer cells" (translation from Latin pathology, which means *the absence of cancer cells' normal abilities to spread and infiltrate other tissues and other organs*).

My contention is that if this had been virtually anything other than cancer, observers to a similar *trial* - meaning the first time a novel method is tested under adequate scientific monitoring by a general practitioner, oncologist, pathologist, surgeons, radiologists – would have ensured that such a *qualitative* result would have led to changes in hospital treatment strategies.

A hospital with respect for itself and their research expertise would probably also have made secondary, *quantitative* studies of the treatment method with regard to whether it is appropriate also for others with the same diagnosis or for patients with other related diagnoses (in our case a second cancer diagnoses).

The journal entries tells that although the GP and oncologist showed positive interest in the method, it had no influence on the Hospital of Vestfold´s (SIV) strategy, which is mainly caused by that cancer treatment are managed centrally from the Norwegian Radium Hospital. It was therefore not made any changes by SIV to standard procedures despite the positively divergent results of the treatment - anomalous compared to *what doctors in advance expected as a result*, namely *that Thoresen treatment would prove ineffective.*

When I myself wanted to draw the only possible logical consequence of this huge deviation from the expected result, this was inexplicable or at least by unexplained reasons strongly opposed by Radium hospital´s side.

My reflection after reading the pages of the diary that describes and documents the facts about this, is that although all the symptoms of active cancer disappeared, the expectation that they would not go away - which can rightly be described as a prejudice – became a guideline for the hospitals' future strategy and the strong recommendations *not* to let the positive facts have any influence on the choice of further treatment.

The indication of this illogical and small research-oriented response from the hospitals side is not meant to show that they generally behave illogically or not research oriented. On the contrary, the intention is to highlight cancer treatments unique position within our health care system and what this form of special status can lead to of undesirable consequences, not only for the individual patient, but also for our health care system and society in general.

I do not draw this conclusion solely on the basis of my initial experiences after the diagnosis, but on the basis of my overall hospital experience. The most obvious adverse experience is presented in the epitome I created from the content in the patient diary - the one that led to the opportunity to undertake a third attempt with Thoresen´s treatment method.

Before we get there, we will briefly return to the second acupuncture treatment - which was necessary because Thoresen had made a mistake in his follow-up control of the energy balance. In the story about the female cancer researcher she conducts her second attempt with the same result as the first. This alludes to that I six months after the first acupuncture treatment with subsequent healing received disturbing symptoms that showed up on the MRI images as a slight growth in the tumor. The reason for this setback Thoresen thought to track using the pulse diagnosis. As mentioned, probably due to an inaccuracy in the follow-up of the disease. After he made an adjustment in the treatment, MRI showed that the small offshoot of the tumor was gone.

The second part of the study is briefly comprised of the following facts:

- Modest growth in tumor detected by MRI after I had a "sensing" that indicated growth.
- Pulse diagnosis, which showed the need for an adjustment of the acupuncture treatment.
- New MRI shortly after a new and slightly modified acupuncture treatment and CT two months later showed that growth for the second time was stopped and the tumor was reduced to the same size as it had previously been.

What I have not included in the story referenced in Chapter 9: "About the laboratory research", is that my acupuncture treatment at a later stage was repeated a third time. It happened almost a year after I had written the story and after hospital checks, this time also including the most advanced diagnostic tools in cancer context, PET CT, indicated that I was healthy and able to live well with an albeit still significant tumor but that did not show growth or contained identified cancer cells[64].

The reason for the second setback is that at best can be described as a medical experiment conducted against my will[65], but which also ended up being the most convincing demonstration of Thoresen treatment method, which until now has been given an adequate qualitative scientific evidence of.

Details before and after the experiment has already been described in Chapter 10 ("Back to the patient diary. An epitome"). You'll just repeat that the growth in a "likely inoperable tumour"[66] was defeated so quickly that an *emergency operation* - to lead the stool through a stoma – was not even applicable.

This brief summary of these dramatic days is the result of a combination of my own notes and hospital records. At no point does these contradict each other. "Probable inoperable tumor" in this context can best be translated as *likely incurable cancer*.

This was the situation when the third part of the qualitative study was conducted by a single one-needle acupuncture treatment to five hundred NoK the same day the disaster was discovered. This part of the study consists of the following components (described in Chapter 9 ["About the laboratory research"]):

• Only a few days after completion of treatment with Avastin PET CT showed strong growth of active cancer cells - where PET CT two months before treatment had not demonstrated any clear pathological situation. Subsequent studies indicated that the remaining cancer cells before treatment were not considered to be pathological, was "triggered" by the treatment to such an extent that they within approximately three months had formed a large and life threatening expiration of the previously pacified main tumour.

• The situation remained unknown to me and therefore untreated by acupuncture during this time because the PET CT images taken immediately after treatment remained in a "drawer". I was therefore not informed about the dramatic change of the illness before I got serious digestive problems and raised the alarm myself.

• The first MRI after the discovery of these fatal errors showed that treatment with Avastin had transformed the situation to likely inoperable (incurable).

• The same day I was informed about the dramatic changes that had occurred immediately after Avastin treatment, I sought out Thoresen, who by pulse diagnosis "read" that the energy balance now was even worse than the first time I was diagnosed.

• Thoresen gave me a new treatment, and I noted significant improvements in the digestive function already in the days following the treatment.

• MRI and CT images taken six months later showed that the growth for the third time was stopped, and that the tumor had shrunk back to the level it had before the Avastin treatment.

oOo

The testing of a new healing method that here is reconstructed, cannot point to an exact statistical significance. However, we get an *indication* of the likelihood that it is the method and not the vagaries that have had an effect on the disease progression for *this one patient*. The probability of this is so overwhelming that no great mathematician in a professional manner will be able to draw it into question.

The next step will be to investigate whether Thoresen´s treatment method is transferable on to other people. Because we cannot yet with 100% certainty know if I'm particularly responsive to this type of treatment, the treatment should be tried on a few more, such as different ages *and in different stages* of the disease. Thus, one can determine if this treatment method has an effect on large populations, or whether it has a more limited scope. In the latter case, one can go a step further and identify limitations. Either way, one will with modest resources have some conclusions on the evidence of the method's efficacy.

My conclusion is that such form of documentation and evidence will give those in charge of our medications and healing methods, a better basis for assessment than the large and hugely expensive, quantitative studies that *some* have demanded. I cannot see another "advantage" of this approval procedure than that it protects the industrial drug production against free competition.

When it comes to *natural cancer treatment*, it lies in the concept that there is not the same risk of negative side effects as there is with chemically manufactured drugs. Though it is in the approval process of naturally developed medications and natural treatment a requirement for documentation related to poisonous substances and mapping of side effects, the acceptance of a qualitative survey will open for a completely different and more free competition, where independent scientists, public hospitals and less private hospitals will be able to afford to attend.

Then the first curative cancer treatment that becomes available, would in no time outperform "the hundred" life-prolonging drugs that are predominant on the cancer drug market today.

14. Statistics as a witness

Analyses indicate that two of the three tumours detected by X-ray, would have disappeared by itself.

Jan Mæhlen, cancer researcher
Dagbladet 27.02.10

I have long been in doubt whether I should convey what authorised cancer treatment has achieved in that time I've had access to statistics. This has several reasons.

It's always more satisfying to convey good news than bad. We've got really good news, and it might be tempted to leave it at that. But given that there is an ambition to give readers an accurate and complete picture of the oncological contemporary Thoresen discovery is born into, it is wrong to exclude the portion of the image that strongly emphasises the need to offer cancer patients an effective curative cancer treatment.

To my surprise, I discovered that the prevailing notions within authorised cancer treatment are far from being the sole within the official health care system. After talking with several cancer researchers I realised that for those who know the conditions, it is an increasingly widespread concern over the lack of treatment efficacy. It has also reached out to the media that more and more believe that *something* should replace the most hazardous drugs. Evidence indicates that the "big" majority are not quite as big as I know most of the alternative therapists believe they are. Therefore, I am no longer quite so worried about being written off as conspiratorial as I feared when I was first considered a project like this.

The conclusions I have drawn in my wandering among both leading and misleading statistics, is also very easy to verify (and more difficult to contradict). Just as knowledge has led us ever more towards natural, renewable sources of energy, I believe especially in the knowledge the statistics convey, and that encourages us to concentrate resources for research on natural cancer treatment to enhance the tumour 's natural tendency to retreat.

Among professionals that conclusion is probably the most controversial, yet the one most difficult to refute. Possibly, Mæhlen is therefore right in that the statement that is reproduced in this chapter's introduction is the result of a "better late than never" mindset. That the prevailing view within authorised cancer treatment are based on assumptions and that we only recently have been able to determine that cancer is dynamic in the sense that they grow and depreciates by circumstances we know *a little* about, though far too little in terms of what is invested of money and time in cancer research.

The reason this is not widely known is that tumours often get unnoticed and disappear without having made us sick - in line with both predictable and unknown factors in our outer and inner life circumstances. This is because they either do not become large before they disappear or are not placed in a cramped place that they press on nerves, or grows in places where they can become large before they are noticed, for example in the stomach/intestines.

It should be mentioned that the senior statistician Zahl at the National Public Health Institute together with Mæhlen are behind the introduction and also stands next to him on the research that has led them and their knowledge forward in the public. This knowledge does not fit into the treatment protocols, at least not what include cancer, which is protected by those who administers consensus. As Moan pointed out to me when he introduced the concept of consensus, it is far from the first time in history that those who manage consensus, are trying to hide the truth.

What we now have of new knowledge about cancer treatment - about vitamin D's significance and more, partly thanks to Moan, Mæhlen and Zahl - and what we have of skills through an effective healing acupuncture method could reverse most of the *last third of the tumours*, those who do not "disappear by themselves" and results in that about a third of the population at some point in their lives suffer from severe cancer.

If we through out lifestyle, i.e. work, leisure, family relationships, social relationships and nutrition - with all that the latter includes of potential poisoning, or too little of basic building blocks for the cells - have come to stimulate the growth of cancer symptom, our thinking and intuition can often lead us to fundamental changes which instead will enhance our own natural ability to influence the disease's withdrawal.

I will give a concrete example that can give an indication of what such a shift in cancer treatment will mean for the individual patient. In this case it regards four living people, two of them admittedly judged moribund and two with very poor statistical prognosis.

Shortly after I had read up on the statistics for the different levels of the progression of the disease, where I was shocked by the death rate for those patients the hospitals failed to heal in the "first round", I received a copy of an email from Switzerland, apparently from one of Thoresen's colleagues, Desirée Oster Wanner. In the mail she tells about four patients she had earlier sent to Thoresen for treatment. All four had shortly after their return reported back to her about their improvement.

When I later, in Chapter 16 ("An evaluation of Thoresen's research") will go through in detail the only study that can give us insight into Thoresen's clinical results, it is important to be aware that an overwhelming majority of those who seek his treatment as a last resort, have cancer at the same stage as these four: the first two with a hundredth parts per thousands and the other two with less than five per cent average chance of survival. It is in this chapter cited the mentioned e-mail together with any future correspondence with Oster Wanner.

By focusing on the central element of natural cancer treatment Thoresen has in all probability *alone* helped more *terminal patients* than all Norwegian cancer wards and hospitals together in the same time period.

While I describe my first contact with a person in Thoresen's international networks through the e-mail from Oster Wanner November 1st 2010, I note that Thoresen has travelled to Nürnberg to lecture about his cancer treatment, and that three weeks earlier he was in Arizona as the main speaker at a congress with participants from all over the United States and with cancer treatment as the main topic. I started to get first hand knowledge of Thoresen's activities and recognition abroad.

I might add that when the book's main editor, PhD. Hans Kolstad, stayed in Switzerland in the winter of 2012, he contacted the person who so far is a professional crown witness of Thoresen's results. He also got a glimpse of how far ahead of Norway Switzerland is with regard to use of acupuncture in the hospitals. Oster Wanner is more than happy to offer her time at our disposal if what has happened in Switzerland, needs to be documented better than the aforementioned e-mail reproduced in this book's appendix.

The more people who report good results, the faster the knowledge of the new view of cancer and the new method of treatment through acupuncture spread throughout the world. Nevertheless, it will go too slow as long as nation like Norway is one of the supporters for the maintenance of the cancer industry's monopoly. The monopoly is protected thru the patent system, the criminalisation of potential competitors and documentation requirements that are so expensive that no one other than the "cartel" has sufficient financial resources to fulfil them.

My claim about the lack of results by authorised cancer treatment is a partial truth. The statistics confirm the extension of life for patients with most types of cancer, and with the high quality of Norwegian cancer hospitals the quality of life for cancer patients in recent decades have also probably been significantly improved. But the main thing, to survive the most prevalent forms of cancer[67], is still as unlikely and doubtful - and just as unpredictable for doctors - as it has been throughout my lifetime and probably generations before that.

The death statistics speak their unique language and allows much of the information conveyed via the media about progress in cancer treatment, at best, can be seen as attempts to create optimism in the population. If this is the goal, it may be justified under the motto "the purpose sanctifies the means": that it is important for cancer patients to go into treatment with belief that it is effective. As a strong supporter of the placebo effect, I agree with this. For the same reason I hesitate to present the correct statistics, which tell the unpleasant truth.

oOo

Before I go into more detail in the statistics, I will quote what medical research has recently discovered about the impact of the most commonly used *antidepressants* used on patients with depression, anxiety, psychosis and a number of related disorders. Initially, I would emphasise that *it is documented efficacy of these drugs in the most severe cases of depression*. The documentation that led to the approval of the medications in the U.S., the EU and a number of other countries, however, *showed that the major user groups concerned they only had an effect on one in four patients*. When medical researchers some decades later now have access to the "negative" parts of the documentation that drug manufacturers weeded out and for several years kept hidden from approving bodies, it turns out that it could not be documented effect on more than one in five subjects[68].

These medications, which only has an effect on a few people within the defined user group has for many years negatively affected four out of five users unnecessarily with the sometimes serious side effects that the use of these medications may cause and also huge costs both for patients and the health budget.

The type of over-medication this is an example of, apply to a variety of medications, especially for the elderly population. However, this widespread practice would be unthinkable in a society where no private financial interest, but patient and public interests has overall responsibility for the development, production and sale of drugs.

I conclude this siding, which is relevant enough in our context, to reiterate that in the case of severely depressed people the antidepressants can both save lives and improve their quality of life.

oOo

If it is as I imagine, that when one has researched for a long time, maybe ones whole life, in a direction that does not provide measurable results outside the lab, and one begins to get an overview which may indicate that there is a different and probably more fruitful direction to investigate, it can be psychologically difficult to accept that this is so. It can also be difficult to believe that a single researcher, mostly alone, but with some help from only one other researcher plus some savings shall be able to succeed with something a whole research community for generations have not succeeded with.

In a sociology historical perspective "mistakes" are changed only after fundamental changes in the prevailing regime. In this case, the error may concern a wrong choice of direction for the research that were taken for more than a century ago. For the medical professionals and political managers that are responsible today such errors can be corrected if it is obvious to many that this is about a mistake.

oOo

After my first and superficial encounters with cancer statistics from the U.S., EU and some Norwegian statistics associated with the mammography discussion I searched deeper into the statistics for Norway. *The Cancer Registry* is the institution in Norway that collects and publishes most of the available Norwegian statistical material in order to present it in an easily understandable form for both professionals, media and the general population. I first went into The Cancer Registry's website and found the statistics entitled "Survival". To my surprise, these statistics showed far better numbers than I had previously seen from other Western countries.

The Cancer Registry´s statistics titled survival goes fifty years back (when this was written - from this year the history is reduced to forty years) and is divided into ten periods. The register shows that there has been significant progress in the so-called *relative survival* (per cent of diagnosed cases), giving an unequivocal impression that modern cancer research and treatment has made similar strides over the past fifty years.

There are large discrepancies, and while I'm going through my own work to find logical errors or miscalculations, I'm finding through internet searches the largest overall statistical survey I have so far had access to. The results of the survey were published in the German Magazine Der Spiegel[69] and is based on 26 years of cancer statistics for Germany from 1978 to 2004. It includes the most common and deadly cancer forms and concluded that there was some greater survival for patients with lung and colorectal cancer, while it was slightly lower for patients with prostate and breast cancer. For all cancers as a whole, there was no significant change. Could the situation really be that much better in Norway?

I have little faith in that, and because I cannot find any reason for the large differences in the figures, I contacted The Cancer Registry by phone. It was the beginning of a dialogue on the telephone and e-mail during a few weeks with statistician and researcher Bjørn Møller, Head of Department at the Registry Division of The Cancer Registry, in order to find the reason(s) for these differences. Møller confirms that cancer treatment is the same in all Western countries. He seems as surprised as me, but have no explanation for the discrepancy. However, his assist by submitting links to expanded figures from the EU.

This is starting to be demanding. Before I get into the new documentation, I decide to review the numbers from Norway and Germany again. I am looking for something that has escaped my gaze, if only a small detail, which in the world of numbers can have serious consequences.

It is something that has escaped my attention, yes most people I would think since all I have so far talked with about the subject, is

202

of the opinion that cancer poses a far smaller risk of death today than just a few years back.

What escaped my attention at the first review of the Norwegian statistics stands as a subtext to the statistics entitled "Survival". There it appears that the statistics is not about how many who survives the disease, but how many people live five years after they were diagnosed. I estimated after using several other statistics that those who die of cancer, on average die about nine years after they were diagnosed, I am left with the feeling of having been thoroughly deceived.

Actually, this statistic tells nothing of interest to most people. For those interested in studying the extension of life, it may be interesting, but only if it is viewed in the context of statistics for a longer period of time. Those who are interested in this, however, would never dream of viewing the only statistics that are titled "Survival". Also, a statistic that told about the development of *lifetime for those who die of the disease*, has a design that would be better suited the purpose.

In my capacity as amateur, but nonetheless representative of the largest user group this publication (website) is intended for, this discovery gave me strong associations with the classic problem of "small print", i.e. formulations whose meaning it is easy to overlook, and that makes one in popular terms, experiencing being deceived.

But where can I find the *true* statistics of survival? The one I can compare the statistics for Germany, which is referred to in Der Spiegel, or with statistics for other countries? I looked and looked but could not find it. It does not exist. I mean, of course it exists, but it's not where most people are looking for it. At just the statistics I was most interested in, is omitted and replaced with a statistic that has the same name as the one we are looking for, makes this even more striking.

When I could not find the right numbers, I had to make statistic myself that showed them. I based it in what I had already made, namely the *average lifetime* of those who die. Then I examined how many had been diagnosed with cancer nine years back (the same as the expected average lifetime), found then the statistics of how many people had cancer on the death certificate nine years later and found that the survival rate is just above one of two.

More precisely I stated that 52.7%[70] of those who get cancer survive.

When one compares The Cancer Registry´s statistics for survival with the statistics for those who actually survive the disease, there are about 63% more people who die from it than the number that The Cancer Registry´s statistics indicate. Available statistics when this was examined in 2013, showed that while The Cancer Registry´s statistics give the impression that the mortality from cancer in Norway in 2010 was reduced to 28.9% of diagnosed cases, the correct statistics show that more than 47% of the diagnosed cases ended up dying of the disease.

I had found the explanation for the discrepancy between the large German study of the changes in survival over 27 years and the Norwegian statistics. The German match well my own figures for Norway, while The Cancer Registry´s statistics are grossly misleading. The alleged strong improvement in survival in the 50 years it's done statistics, does not apply to survival, but the extension of life of the patients who ends up dying from the disease. A first conclusion is thus that cancer research has succeeded in giving patients several years of life, but it has failed to develop curative treatment, with the exception of some less common cancers, which have no bearing on the overall picture.

After an initial telephone conversation with Møller and some general approaches to the problem from my side by e-mail I could now report back on my findings.

I got the following answer:

> ... I agree that five-year survival does not give the whole picture, especially for cancers that can relapse even after 15 and 20 years ...

The first part of the answer was fine, but the last part of the sentence brought me to new uncertainties. That it is described as a relapse if you are getting cancer 15 and 20 years after first getting diagnosed and have been without symptoms for many of those years, I can understand. But it cannot in my view be described as a relapse if you have been sick and/or under treatment in a large part of this time.

Current statistics regards surviving patients as those who are still under treatment after five years. Therefore, it is totally wrong to suggest that they then die by a relapse if they for instance die after six, seven or eight years. Even if they were to die of cancer five years and a few days after they are diagnosed, they are on the statistics as survivors.

Another question is whether it should be characterised as relapse in case you get a new symptom outbreak and die of the same cancer. A general judgment indicates that although the disease symptoms are removed by chemotherapy, surgery and radiation and not immediately afterwards come back again, it is still wrong to say that the disease is cured if the patient later dies of the same type of cancer.

The cancer patients I have described here, dying of the disease after five years and does not "fit" in this type of statistics, will paradoxically enough, be on the same statistics at least twice. First as cured in case they are still alive five years after diagnosis. If they recover after more than five years and then get a relapse and die within a further period of five years, they are automatically registered again, but now with opposite sign. However, if they relapse and survive another five years, they will a second time be a possible false positive entry in the statistics, which theoretically may have more false positive five-year periods. Looking at the numbers of breast cancer survivors, we find that, on average, they die almost 13 years after diagnosis[71]. Hence, a large number of these appear at least twice in statistics as false positive cases.

That the statistics of survival for five years testifies a steady percentage increase over the past fifty years shows as mentioned no increase in survival from the disease, but an extension of life of those who ends up dying from the disease. Statistics become, in other words increasingly misleading as new drugs prolong lifetime. If this is the way to keep statistics continue in the years ahead, we are approaching a situation where only about half as many actually survive cancer as The Cancer Registry reports.

Aside from the obvious economic motives among private providers in the health sector, whether for equipment or medications, I have been careful not to speculate on the motives behind the reprehensible conditions in cancer research and treatment. When I brought up the results of my statistical calculations with one of the cancer researchers I have sought knowledge and advice from, Jan Mæhlen, I suggested that the misleading statistic originally was far more accurate than it is now, as it was designed at a time when lifetime (fifty years ago) was significantly shorter than today. Because I first had seen an exact similar statistics from the U.S., I would add that it may originally have been just copied from there in order to have a statistical basis for comparison. But before I finished my attempt to "whitewash" The Cancer Registry - which was because I had never come up with the idea that such deliberate manipulation could occur in small, honourable Norway -, I was interrupted - by Mæhlen, who had previously been employed in The Cancer Registry and as I have already written, he confirmed that this is really about fraud, with obvious economic motives.

In one of my subsequent web searches to try to find out if something was published about this profession secret, I found nothing for Norway. However, I came across an interesting contribution on You Tube by Dr. Leonard Coldwell, an American specialist in stress-related illnesses, where he, as the only one so far I have seen, who speaks of how the population and politicians are deceived by the cancer statistics for survival. In addition, he had news that made this phenomenon even spicier. There recently has in fact been changes made to the statistics for survival in the United States. These changes are so brazen that it is strange that not central, neutral media has discovered it. The change consists in that *the fifth year is removed*. The consequence of that statistic now portrays it as if patients survive the disease if they are still alive four years after they were diagnosed, is that it gives the impression of an amazing progress in cancer treatment effectiveness from one year to the next.

I understand the quoted researcher's frustration in the way that new breakthroughs in cancer research indirectly is undermined by those who have the power to make definitions. By presenting misleading statistics through the years have given the impression that cancer research is making progress and has thus stopped a legitimate demand from the public about actions by politicians for a revision and amendment of our cancer care.

Meanwhile, the latest news from the United States reinforced what I regard as the Americanisation of Norwegian health care system, although The Cancer Registry has at least not yet dared to copy the "stunt" from the American Cancer Society. Unless they change the statistics to define "survival for four years" before this present book is published.

They have however ventured something I think is even worse, as seen from a legal point of view. When I during the last edit made a deeper scrutiny of their other publications, it was in fact clear that presenting misleading information is not limited to the aforementioned statistics. The Cancer Registry has also in its yearbook presented completely wrong conclusions regarding progress in mortality. If it is true what the researcher claimed that those working with this are intentionally keeping us in the dark, then The Cancer Registry Statics take a major step towards an action I would think puts you under the Penal Code. The statistics can possibly be justified by what is written in "small print". What I found in the yearbook *Cancer in Norway 2010*, the chapter "Trends in Incidence, Mortality and Survival of cancer in Norway 1966-2010" published on The Cancer Registry´s website is harder to explain away. This chapter describes mistakenly significant progress with regard to the survival of the disease. The author(s) use here the mentioned statistics of survival after five years *as if they actually provide a true picture of the changes in the survival of the disease*[72]. Disinformation is spread through the yearbook in a way that can not be explained away. The conclusions it presents is the opposite of what is actually the case: The annual report states that there has been a significant improvement in mortality for cancers where *the truth is that there has been no significant improvement in mortality over the last fifty years*. For most of the cancer diseases.

It was only when I had made this discovery, and my involvement in cancer statistics had come to an end, I began to suspect why for more than a decade it has been possible to arrive at diametrically opposite conclusions on the issue if mammography screening reduces or increases mortality from breast cancer.

Because this is on the edge of my main focus, I have not had the capacity to scrutinise the respective studies presented, but in that The Cancer Registry both organised mammography screening and also has completely misleading statistics for survival of breast cancer, I do not rule out that this may be about a serious source of error, which in turn leads to another and equally serious error. It would not surprise me if Mæhlen and Zahl too had this as the basis of their studies of the mammography problem.

In the perspective of what new research and knowledge about natural healing, the extensive figures I have undergone from the United States, European Union, Germany and Norway, which covers a period of fifty years, has given me some surprises. In view of these facts, I have made up the following status:

> • Advances in cancer research and treatment in the Western world over the past fifty years has led to a significant improvement in the time between diagnosis and death date.
> • In the same period there has been significant improvement in survival for some less common cancers.
> • Modern cancer research and treatment has not led to significant improvement in the survival of cancer diseases generally considered in the last fifty years.

• New findings confirm cancer´s dynamic character and that an estimated two out of three tumours diminish by itself through self healing.

• Cancer´s dynamic character leads to the question whether the current treatment, with some exceptions, statistically gives better results than no treatment. This doubt is due to the knowledge of the disease´s dynamic nature and low discovery of the disease in the natural societies without cancer hospitals. Likewise, more cancer patients than previously seeking lifestyle changes and strategies that strengthen the immune system express it.

• For advanced cancer, there is a statistically low probability of survival by authorised cancer treatment that will not result in any significant increase in mortality risk choosing a treatment that aims to strengthen the energy of life and improve quality of life, rather than continue a costly treatment that weakens both. On the other hand it seems that different forms of *natural cancer treatment* increase the prospect of survival for cancer patients today termed *terminal*.

The last point concerns tens of thousands of Norwegians today, equivalent to a medium-sized Norwegian city. Any real (legal) treatment option for this group is not available in Norway and most other Western countries. If at some point it becomes possible for severely affected cancer patients to choose a life invigorating and possible curative treatment when authorised treatment is unsuccessful and prognosis of survival are minimal, it is essential that the different involved clinicians can work together.

I have not found any objective reason why such cooperation is non-existent and to me it seems to be systematically opposed by "the system" - but motivated by subjective interests. How far we currently are from cooperation, especially with regard to the terminal patient´s survival probability, you can find examples of in the book's epilogue "From the political highest level".

It has been a sad affair to be the one who by chance discovered the apparent large discrepancy between the survival rates of cancer in Norway and Germany, and then the reason for this disparity.

Given that I have mentioned the help I got to figure this out by Møller from The Cancer Registry, I end this chapter with my impressions after a telephone and e-mail dialogue with Møller autumn 2010.

Towards me Møller was genuinely helpful, and he seemed credible when he did not understand what the difference between Germany and Norway consisted in. Anyway, I will not pass characteristics, and the last thing I want to risk, is to strike at individuals who have made mistakes because they themselves are victims of an integrated system failure. It is those who know what is done wrong and have the power to change the conditions, which I now want to come in dialogue with - not to criticise, but to achieve change. If Møller has such power, I believe indeed that a dialogue in connection with the publication can lead to change.

I have read a broad discussion about Møller´s doctorate, where he seems critically to get behind The Cancer Registry's long tradition of false claims of great progress in cancer treatment in terms of survival. The featured story in the discussion of the doctoral degree indicates that Møller stands for the opposite, that he relates to the true figures for the survival of cancer and presents an unvarnished picture of the state of affairs. This is shown by Møller´s conclusion, consisting of a prognosis where the increase in the number of cancer incidents from 1997 to 2020 (23 years) is estimated to be just below 40%. Because we have the gold standard backward from 1997 to 1958 (39 years), where we have had an increase of 60%, we see a future still weak, rising curve toward the not too distant future where cancer diseases may prove to be one even greater threat to the survival of our civilisation than climate change. Seen from a realist point of view, it is precisely the rise in the curve that makes such fears justified. Although the climb is weak one must take into consideration the already high level of mortality. And considering that the prognosis of mortality from the disease do not show significant improvement, it is in my view just as naive[73] to think that our cancer research will address this, at some time in our children's future - as the belief that our technological development to stop the warming of our atmosphere.

This fact makes Møller and I to probably fully share the view of the urgent need to develop an offer with curative cancer treatment.

The next chapter contains some considerations of ethics and economics, which all in all has given me a new and much more negative view of our world and the organisation of society than I had when I started this work. I thought I had versatile life experience, including business and finance. However, it has been shown that it was not versatile enough and that I also had an overly naive belief that the health care system is an exception in an otherwise money- and power-driven civilisation - at least, in the outer and material sense.

The following book pages I will go further in exemplification of what I am referring to, which still betrays a naive believe that at some point, for man of important context comes the crucial turning point: that we in Norway show that we are serious about human rights - including the right to the best available treatment for health issues - precedes all other considerations.

15. Ethics and economics in cancer treatment

Ethics is known as one of the main disciplines of philosophy. Just as the discipline medicine rightfully demand respect for own professionalism and expertise this requirement applies also to other scientific disciplines. In this case, it is the subject ethics I will defend - because ethics is one of the disciplines most often mixed with other subjects in an unprofessional way.

The paradox is that using ethics for such purposes is fundamental unethical. Ethics is like mathematics an absolute, in regards to that for example lying in a given situation is equally reprehensive for everybody and not something that can be manipulated by some or put up against anything else. Together with medical science ethics forms an especially important combination of subjects. Simply because the latter always is about human life and welfare. However, I had not believed that this combination could have negative sides, until I began to look for reasons why the chemical and high-tech pharmaceutical industry's monopoly in cancer treatment have arisen and have been preserved over more than a century in a world where market forces is the ideal, free competition is legal and cartels are punishable.

Strangely enough the cancer treatment monopoly in almost all Western liberal democracies is enforced so hard that it is prohibited and punishable for competitors to offer their services. In many Western countries, unauthorised or alternative healthcare therapists expose themselves for jail time if they offer cancer patients help - regardless of whether they have harmed or helped the patient.

Before the new law of 2003, a lifesaver as Thoresen risked prosecution, sentence and imprisonment for having healed terminal cancer patients. However, he avoided further prosecution and any sentence since he was reported after 2003.

How can it be that at some point in the early twentieth century it was widely prevalent considered ethically reprehensible for unauthorised medical professionals to help people with cancer to be freed from the disease? Not only reprehensible, but directly criminal, and to such an extent that it could trigger vast imprisonment?

Where does this dogma come from? And how can it be that the highest courts in the world's most advanced law states have accepted such a legally considered very "loose" claim?

Eventually I came to the conclusion that the medical basis for using ethics in this context is based on the same "loosely" reasoned dogma that cancer is an irreversible disease that can not be treated effectively in any other way than through the services the cancer treatment´s monopoly supply. That it is a dogma, have previously been confirmed by one of the country's most prominent cancer researchers, the aforementioned Jan Mæhlen, who confirmed that no cancer research supports this hypothesis. Nor is there any possible scientific explanation for it, as it already is belied by the facts. All research in this area, still according to Mæhlen, shows just the opposite, that cancer is a reversible disease, which constantly heals naturally by self-healing.

An important question is why such crucial knowledge about the disease has not previously been explored and clarified. Why has this not been medically interesting enough to be further investigated?

The answer has hardly anything to do with science, or lack of medical interest. It is more natural to seek the cause in the fact that those who primarily pay for research do not want their scientists to "see" in the direction where cancer is cured naturally. The reason is that what the researchers will then be able to find both can weaken the monopoly and reduce the "market" - the number of cancer patients over time. By mapping this area and the organism's own defences against cancer, will probably sooner or later lead to methods to strengthen or restore the organism's natural defences against cancer. This will of course be a major breakthrough in cancer research, yet also pose a great threat to those who today are suppliers of the services in the world´s cancer care.

Another and probably equally important prerequisite for the maintenance of the monopoly is the huge financial requirements for those who can demonstrate promising research into new medication. These requirements are based *in the way* the medication´s effect are required documented, a process that is so costly to implement that even nation-states like Norway has not seen themselves financially able to compete with the cancer drug industry. That we do so even on the basis of purely medical motives, but then as soon as something interesting is discovered, instead see ourselves forced to sell out to large corporations with purely economic motives, this has so far only had negative consequences for the cancer patients that I have so far tried to clarify.

Also, much of what was originally discovered and researched within alternative medicine and are considered to be of commercial interest to the major drug companies, sooner or later ends in the process being acquired by one of the major manufacturers. If it is effective in a way that it threatens the market it is not surprising that it is purchased in order *not to be* further studied, so it can be developed into a patented drug. Those who originally stood for the good ideas and the first part of the research are powerless in relation to such a decision and must passively witness a lid put on their discovery. Here the majority dictatorship applies and those with majority shareholding are in charge. Their discovery is bought and paid for by the company as if they actively oppose the decision of investigating further or go into partnership with other players, they are effectively stopped by a law that absolutely should not be used to select the type of cancer medication we are offered.

In summary, I believe to have seen and described a simple, efficient and highly profitable business mechanism that protects the economically strongest players, but that has nothing to do with medicine and human welfare.

The most strange phenomenon to me in this "organisation" is that the major parties in this, manufacturers and the health authorities that regulate the conditions for letting anyone into the market has worked together so well and for so long to increase the development costs - with an initial result preventing smaller operators' access to the market. Secondly the health bureaucracy and politicians give the other party – the major manufacturers, which has the market to themselves - all profits on the taxpayers and patients' expense.

oOo

So far, I wanted to show how basic ethical and economic principles, to some extent, legal, is used and abused in two-or three-team to earn a small group of investors' interests. In one case medical assessments are also involved, in some cases also a crucial prerequisite for investors so far experiencing phama-stocks as safe placements.

The thesis that symptom destruction is the only form of cancer treatment that could save the patient's life, is essential to the *link*[74] between ethics, economics, law and medicine that has upset me the most. Here it is the link between this medical dogma and the concept of "false hope" that has cleared the way for the criminalisation of anyone who offers cancer patients a different form of treatment.

In this is a paternalistic attitude and pompous prejudge: Those who have the power to define, pretending *to know with certainty* that no one else is or will be able to help cancer patients. With reference to the earlier-quoted principle of scientific research that was originally put forward by Popper (described in conversation with Manzetti in Chapter 11), a hypothesis that no one but I can help cancer patients - without this claim on all known methods is tested falsified – is anti-scientific in its nature. It is then also further toward a field not aiming at scientific results but to maximise profits. If a scientific attitude had been the guide it would have been placed the greatest importance to examine whether the hypothesis is correct, i.e. that there are other avenues of research, such as in alternative and other cultures medicine that could provide equal or better results compared to western medical science.

If our cancer care had been primarily medical science motivated, and remained as acclaimed science theory assumes,

Thoresen´s clinical results would at least ten years ago have been met with medical curiosity and followed up with thorough scientific investigation rather than first being tried "silenced to death" - without investigating the effect of the method of treatment - and then, when in 2013 it was approached such an investigation was actively opposed.

What happened in the latter, will be elucidated in the book's epilogue which refers a number of extraordinary events in connection with that the public, by Telemark University College, after the initiative of a Ph.D. student, was trying to conduct a scientific study of the effects Thoresen´s treatment has on dogs.

A good illustration of some of the collective ingrained prejudices associated with the cancer issue is what happened when Manzetti sent files with his research material to a colleague he had studied with, and who now found himself *within* the Radium hospital´s tall research-walls. The next day this answer came:

> We know that acupuncture has no effect on cancer, so we have no time to look at this.

Instead of going further into the jungle of unscientific or anti-scientific prejudices and statements filed by people who claim to represent Scientific truth itself (as if they fought with God on their side) - I will dwell by the following statement, namely that anyone other than authorised physicians (God's elect) who tries to interferer with the cancer treatment market giving patients false hope. This form of fighting competitors to the monopoly is particularly worrisome when it comes to cancer patients that hospitals no longer have nothing but pain relief to offer - before death.

False hopes is a term that initially appears to be slightly negative, in this context, something reprehensible, but that linguistically is considered an oxymoron. False hopes do not exist. Either the patient has hope - or not.

However, there is no doubt that *someone* has sought to describe *something* as so immoral that it should be prohibited. Regardless if the intention was to protect the monopoly it became the

216

result when the lawmakers confident that the medical assessment is scientific substantiated, has forbidden a diverse group of health professionals to help the *terminal* cancer patients. Those who once long ago launched the claim that none other than cancer wards in hospitals can help cancer patients, and *especially when hospitals are realising that they can not help them*, has gotten a well-trained health care system, judiciary, politicians and legislators to first accept that "false hope" exists, and secondly, without having submitted any scientific evidence also achieved that virtually all the other citizens, including legislators, thinking that this was a fact[75].

What most of us for generations have believed in has paradoxically been strongest fortified in the course of the disease where it should have been the most clear that authorised treatment are not alone in being able to help cancer patients, namely in the stage where doctors tell patients (and others) that they can not help and therefore denotes those as dying. That the patient is dyeing as the last information, is both wrong and unethical - and an indirect admission that they have *never* helped the patient with the disease (as it is stated that they will die from it). As an additional admission[76] it is putting additional authority behind the statement that the patient is dying by a new claim regarding the patients' remaining lifetime.

Losing hope means the opposite of placebo. *Nocebo* is a mentally applied health destructive impulse. To inflict nocebo is unethical and after what I can understand an almost inevitable consequence of a doctor with the authority his position comes with claims that the patient can not recover *because the same doctor is unable to help the patient get well*.

Lothar Hirnreises research (ref. note 76) is essentially a voluminous documentation that it is many different and many others who can help and demonstrably helped a large number of patients who have had their death sentence by hospital doctors[77]. It is a statistically high percentage of those few patients who have resisted the nocebo, it means to be notified of his imminent death, who have maintained *genuine hope*, taken responsibility for their lives and taken initiative to become healthy again - and survives!

oOo

Almost the whole world has accepted the concept of false hope and the way the concept within medicine, ethics, law and ultimately economics has been used, I envision this as perhaps the most successful example of collective *brainwashing* that we can find and also should be able to agree on, if we make a scientific investigation of this from a historical and sociological perspective.

I now also use the subjects sociology and history, including contemporary history, this is because the problems that are associated with cancer diseases require an extended perspective to find a good solution for the future, and preferably contemporary cancer patients as well.

The reason I use the term brainwashing, is my own sense of having been subjected to it myself. Before I started this book project, I thought that medicine was such an important matter that behind medical progress in our Western health care system were public and neutral, professional drivers. The truth is that most of the drugs we buy, is the result of commissioned research on order by a few of the world's largest chemical industrial corporations. I thought that we - by our elected leaders - who ordered the medications we need most to develop. Now I have learned that it is the reverse: that it is we - the research groups and the public - who are the servants of purely private interests[78].

How the industry has successfully managed to turn this relationship upside down, while most of us are not even aware that it happened, or has accepted, is due to a subject that is about as far away from the art of healing one can get, namely *marketing*. This is not marketing, as we ordinary consumers know from daily life. It is marketing aimed at two professions: the medical and the legal. Moreover, it is aimed towards nation-states represented by their officers, politicians, ministries and governments. The purpose of the promotion was, and still is, according to those I have talked to and who have avoided being caught by it, to establish a pipeline into nation states' treasuries.

This is a type of marketing we would not have accepted if we had been aware of it and its ultimate goal. Many people have probably heard of an American marketing technique that consists in alluring product images are inserted in commercials or television programs, in which brief moments that our conscious perception does not detect them. Yet they are seen and affects us subconsciously[79].

The marketing I am referring to is something completely different, but have in common with the aforementioned U.S. television commercial that it affects us without us being aware of it or know how. For this reason it should be banned. The great paradox when it comes to stealth marketing, however, is: *How to forbid something going on behind our backs?*

In the link below note 76 shows a number of examples of how influencing consciousness through television images that have either well hidden messages or exposed in such short span of time that our waking consciousness can not see them, while they still affect our trade patterns so strongly that this is a profitable strategy.

The specific example I will describe is already described in the previous chapter as deliberate manipulation of statistics. A technique that is also developed in the U.S., especially for the cancer industry and already many decades ago adopted by The Cancer Registry, which although they do not have products to sell has its own and other Norwegian cancer researcher existence within medicine to defend.

The marketing has successfully got us to believe in the manufactured drugs and they keep getting better, but it primarily serves manufacturers by expanding the market for medications, increase profits and falsely lure with greater possibility of survival. Isolated cases of lasting recovery are highlighted in the media with immediate massive pressure for new grants, while for most drugs concerned, it is about prolonged residual life and increased consumption of the most expensive medications.

Is this just the tip of the iceberg? Does the marketing rely on cold calculation and manipulation that is hidden under the surface and that can be the basis for more advanced forms of marketing we have not yet discovered? Of course it was not intended that the above manipulation of television and film images would be revealed. It would have probably not been discovered if none that had a hand in any of those examples, chose a more reputable profession and leaked information through critical journalism.

The possibility exists that other marketers, such as ones with assignments for the cancer industry has been better with secrecy, so that neither doctors, patients, families, cancer researchers, health bureaucrats, politicians, journalists and the wider layers of the population has discovered that, contrary to wanting to help those affected by cancer, the cancer industry's real objective is the opposite, namely to increase the market and the flow in the "straws" or pipelines they have drilled into state funds to countries with public health care system[80].

My hypothesis is that European countries have been caught off guard by getting conclusions that just apparently have been the results of proper professional and democratic processes in the United States, but which in reality is the result of processes we in Scandinavia and Norway are little familiar with and probably also would not accept from our elected decision makers' side.

There are a wide variety of examples in the United States of collusion between private interests and private interest groups on the one hand and public administration and politics on the other. To prove this claim can best be done by referring to *Sicko*, the award-winning film with documentary filmmaker Michael Moore's unchallenged claims about America's health care system. Here we see a large number of the most influential politicians in both the Democratic and Republican side, parading past the camera with an attached price tag that says how much they get paid on top of their regular salary in the form of a bonus from the pharmaceutical industry. In Norway, this would be judged as corruption, while in the United States is an accepted part of politicians "lobbying", part of an incorporated (un)culture that provides the greatest economic operators greater academic, administrative and political influence than in any other democratic countries.

220

The film Sicko has made many Norwegians aware of the major differences between American and Scandinavian healthcare. It can also give us insight into aspects of health care we have inherited without actually having undertaken an independent analysis of it or considered if it is the way we want it to be.

It is not unlikely that these payments to politicians are recognised as expenses for marketing. A prime example of successful "marketing", which I assume is due to paid political supporters, is the claim that it is ethically reprehensible for alternative therapists to give cancer patients hope that the disease can be stopped. This was in turn the reasoning to introduce legislation that punishes this "crime" by fines and in serious cases also with imprisonment. That this has succeeded in U.S., is understandable with the money "persuasion". I'm more surprised of the successful import of this model to Scandinavia and Norway in a way that has resulted in our medical and legal professionals and the majority of our elected policy makers at the time circumvent the normal legal accepted forms of evidence, such as witness statements, witnessed condition reports, photographs, film, etc., and vouched for an argument without root in medical or legal professionalism.

The first examples of this that I have come across is from talented, but also at times brutal marketers who early in the last century helped the U.S. chemical drug industry to emerge victorious out of several matches against alternative medical directions, including a very promising development of electromagnetic medicine in the early 1900s, which ended up being banned.

So it is from the United States and throughout more than a century of practice we know the methods to ban the losing party to practice their treatment methods, and to imprison players who would not bow to political regulations and new laws, but who continued to fight for medical strategies they themselves considered as academically superior. Those who lacked financial backers, who could have made the fight fair, often lost everything.

It is still made movies and books about this unflattering prehistory to the U.S. health care system. One of those who have studied this field inbound and published information in articles and books, is the Norwegian doctor Vilhelm Schjelderup (see bibliography at Wikipedia). Partly because of this mediation, I believe, he has also been subjected to persecution in Norway from many of his colleagues and from the health care authorities.

There is much within this and other areas of American and "Americanised" European health care systems that could be cited under the heading "Ethics and Economics". However, I will limit myself to a particular case from the news (in 2011) which I consider to be a good example of the commercial for *the American ways* penetration in European countries' health policies.

May 2nd 2011 a new EU directive was introduced which prohibited the sale of all herbal medications until they eventually had obtained new approval. There were also major limitations in the sale and marketing of natural remedies and supplements.

The "advertisement" for the directive stipulates *that the regulations will provide better information to the consumer*. Possibly there is some truth in this, which of course is a good intention if it had been a probability that this and not very different consequences of the directive was intended by those who originally planted the seed for this radical intervention in the health care market.

I have no doubt that the directive's European proponents believe in the "advertisement", but I doubt they know the origin and why it has for many years been running a vigorous campaign for this directive.

I will stick to the facts and prognostics presented on NRK P2 when I show examples of how the new regime distorts the current competitive situation in favour of the largest pharmaceutical manufacturers and large pharmacy chains and results in adverse consequences for consumers. The consequences that really has meaning, has nothing to do with "better information to consumers". No advance publicity is run for the radical restriction of the so-called alternative market participants *freedom of action* (in the best sense). It is the legal ideal of free market the directive fundamentally undermines and had it not been for some independent press, as the society newsroom in NRK P2, very few consumers, if any, would have been familiar with what was planned before it was adopted .

For me, which on the basis of my own cancer began to interest me for market mechanisms in the health industry, and especially for the kind of cancer medications that are predominant on the market, the introduction of the EU directive is a daily example of how monopolies and cartels could arise in the past. This time it's the "alternative part" of the market to be taken over by those who after the directive´s commencement afford to meet its requirements, and how those who are least economically interesting, and those that are interesting but do not want to sell, is "regulated "out of the market. Nevertheless, one can expect that the latter group will be able to come back on the market with a new name and some cosmetic changes, making it difficult for them to reach forward with legal action against the parties who stole their product. At best, they are awarded compensation that under no circumstances replace the loss of a business and the jobs it represents.

The consequence of the directive in cold facts shows that Germany[81] lost 93% of the market overnight with 14,000 jobs. 9,300 natural medications should be taken down from the shelves on a permanent basis - notably if the players follow the new directive. The 7% of the products that survives this restructuring is essentially directly or indirectly produced by the chemical drug industry. I ask myself if there really are any, be they politicians, bureaucrats, medical or other, which, after thinking twice about it, believe that this will be for the benefit of public health in Germany and is truly done for the sake of the patients?

Most of these natural medications are not introduced in the small and already stringent Norwegian market. Here it is primarily the *natural preparations* (natural extracts with people medically recognised effect against various health problems) and *dietary supplements* (including vitamins and minerals) that is affected by making it illegal to promote the purpose of the product. In practice, this will not only mean financial disaster for most of the health food manufacturers and vendors. Thanks to this strike at free speech, the EU directive is a threat to the preservation of folk medical trivia, a priceless treasure that is kept alive by the part of the health industry that the directive touches - if not the resistance against it proves to be so strong that it is not enforced.

Moreover, one can ask what are the long term consequences of the government now criminalising the sales and marketing of natural medications and supplements that large parts of Europe's population uses. I feel pretty sure that the purpose of the directive is to stop a long trend of transition from chemist to health food products, a development caused by *the patients' subjective experience of that natural preparations are good, and that these give them better health and quality of life. Removing preparations from the shelves will consequently have to lead to poorer health and quality of life and to varying degrees mean that they must be replaced by both more economically and medically intensive medication.*

For many years, natural and folk medicine had such a steady growth that statisticians and forecasters have long since seen that it is only a matter of when it would begin to "steal" significant market share from the chemical drug industry. The EU directive can be seen as the clearest sign that the battle about what kind of medication that will be dominant in the future of health care, is seriously running. With the directive the chemical industry has increased its lead and differential treatment in favour of themselves on the formal area. It remains to be seen how patients and sellers of natural medications react to the new prohibition of sales, and if the population's increasing use of natural medications, natural remedies and dietary supplements can be suppressed.

oOo

Below I mention some facts (in italics) followed by my subjective thoughts of how ethics is used in unethical behaviour:

> • *It is prohibited to market products that support natural cancer treatment unless the information for the product is scientifically proven.*

224

Comment: It is not acceptable with the type of evidence that is good enough for legal adjudication, but only one type of evidence that is so expensive to establish that in practice only the pharmaceutical industry can afford it. If the intent is the one given by the health authorities, namely to ensure patients the right information about natural medicine and supplements, there is in my view other and better ways to do it than to introduce a ban that effectively deprives patients the possibility of using these herbal products and - medications.

• *It is illegal and punishable for non-authorised health professionals to give cancer patients hope of recovery. In the context of the EU directive this will reduce the possibility of reaching patients with natural medicine and supplements that can strengthen their ability to fight the disease themselves.*

Comment: As known, one does not need to be a doctor to know that giving a terminally ill patient hope for improvement - true or false – gives a better the prognosis for recovery than no hope. Criminalising both therapists, marketers and sellers of natural medicines and dietary supplements are an exceptionally effective combination if their objective is to close the monopolist competitors out in the cold. If we add that the consequences of a death sentence on those patients hospitals can not provide life-saving treatment for leads to abandonment and reduced interest to try a cure, we get a situation where the current legislation leads to that even larger amounts of expensive life-prolonging drugs are sold, and less affordable natural and life-strengthening drugs.

• *A comprehensive Canadian study conducted on 1,179 women in Nebraska (USA) over four years shows that optimisation of the population's vitamin D intake will reduce the incidence of cancer to less than a quarter of today. The Health Bureaucracy in the United States immediately dismissed the results of the study. Later, other*

225

*Western countries followed the United States and decided to
focus on what may help to cast doubt on the study, by
warning the population that large doses of vitamin D can be
harmful.*

Comment: The "alleged hazard" the health
authorities will protect the population against, can not
possibly be near the dangers of getting cancer. A few hours
in the sun in a Norwegian summer gives us namely up to 50
times the vitamin D content in the blood that are currently
recommended by health authorities, and 20 times that which
was given to subjects in the Nebraska study. I've never heard
of anyone who has had side effects of such a "massive
overdose" as a Norwegian summer in good weather,
according to the latest reviews the health authorities can
provide.

In contrast to the studies the drug industry finances,
the Nebraska study is *independent*[82], as is the case for most
other vitamin D studies. This means that they at least can not
be suspected of having financial motives for putting vitamin
D in a particularly favourable light. Moreover, the Nebraska
study is based on experiments with multiply the number of
people compared to what is considered sufficient[83] for what
the drugs may undergo for the final testing on large
populations.

In other words, the health care authorities demand
better scientific evidence to adjust the population's intake of
vitamin D to the level the Nebraska study shows can remove
up to three out of four cases of cancer than is required to
allow toxic and highly health-depleting cancer medicine on
the Norwegian population. This is not only difficult to
understand. It is impossible to accept.

• *The general attitude within the authorised cancer
treatment is that it is not sufficient evidence of the link
between diet and cancer. For this reason, nutritional
physiology - possibly because this is considered to provide
cancer patients false hope of recovery - not included in*

treatment strategies in Norwegian hospitals. Only recently, information on nutrition physiology is applied in a simple brochure that can be taken home.

Comment: Around the 10 000 independent studies[84] that are designed to detect associations between food (in the broadest sense, what we take in) and cancer is not considered sufficient evidence that there are such relationships and this has as yet not led to patients being given clear recommendations about what one should and should not eat and drink. This viewpoint is not a backlog of "old days" but has recently been advocated by a health professional authority, leader of the Norwegian Oncological Association, Andreas Stensvold[85].

oOo

That lack of ethics leads to a lot of money in a few hands, mentioned in an earlier footnote (76). We understand perhaps better the amount of 1200 billion crowns - the major drug producers' profits - when it illustrates that the largest U.S. pharmaceutical manufacturers' profits are in the order of ten times the Norwegian health budget. If we estimate that they have a net profit of 10% of turnover, when it is sold annually American drugs at a gross cost of the nations that buy equivalent to one hundred Norwegian health budgets. Considering the western countries' overuse of chemical medications we can talk about huge savings if marginally useful and directly harmful medications, which in turn creates new markets for the increasing number of drugs for individual patients, are replaced with strategies and medications that strengthen the human nature´s innate capacity for self-healing.

A summary of the financial aspects must necessarily be generalisations and conclusions are primarily intended as food for thought, not as definitive statements.

• Most medical research centres in the Western countries are developing the products that the owners of the largest transnational drug manufacturers believe their companies are best served by producing.

• Drugs that scientists, doctors and health authorities would have preferred to give patients, are only produced in those cases where the patient interests coincide with the producers' economic interests.

• The public authorities will develop sales channels for drug manufacturers through their respective approval procedures. However, these principles follow in the American model. They favour the largest producers and discriminate their competitors through stringent demands for evidence for the effect of the medication. (Cf. the ever stronger restrictions on the sale and marketing of natural medication and medical supplements in the EU / EEA.)

• The governments buy the industry's products over their budgets and recommends the country's doctors to recommend their patients to buy them, either by their own money or grants from various government schemes.

      With some exceptions, the public pays the price the producers themselves set, although the production is based on patents and consequently with no price competition. By their calculations and accounts the producers show to large differences between prices and costs. Generally it is considered unproblematic in ethical context that the investor gets an extra return for taking a risk. Regarding medications the patents, monopoly and cartel activities contribute to that the risk is less and the returns higher than what is normal in business. This is notably concerning the major drug manufacturers, which have long been major and the ownership extending over generations. For the little ones who want to enter among the great, as Norwegian Clavis Pharma, the jungle laws is still valid. They have similar negligible impact on national health budgets.

• When *recommending* to a patient and in many cases requiring the patient to buy a special medication - something I have experienced myself: *"unless you try this medication, I can not still give you sick-leave"* - the doctor gets an extra income. For the seconds it takes to write out a prescription, the doctor receives a bonus in addition to payment for the consultation. It is in principle a double payment. It's not big, but the scheme illustrates a system where the players' profits are entangled in professional decisions in a way that allows me to associate the concept of legalised and systematic corruption, albeit on a small scale and negligible volume compared to the aforementioned corruption in the health market in USA. This is about the principle and the far from negligible consequences in the extension of it: At one end of this "food chain" the patient risks being over- or wrongly medicated. At the other end the doctor and all the subsections from drug production to distribution and sales are left with an unreasonably high profit on the patient's (health) and community's (economic) cost.

We live in an age where online research and nanotechnology has produced everyday products that are so advanced that only their inventors understand how this is possible. The same generation accepts to be transported around using 150 year old technology (ineffective explosion engines in spite of recent decades major improvements), where most of the energy is wasted as heat, while polluting our communities and is one of the largest threats to human survival on earth. At the same time these engines empty the bearings of possibly one of our most valuable non-renewable natural resources.

Just as the oil industry cartels that once divided the world's oil wealth among themselves, which alone determines the price (OPEC) and until further notice almost succeeded in stopping the development of new technologies that in all respects would be beneficial for both users and earth – i.e. for all but those who own the oil companies - the chemical cancer industry has succeed with a similar "piece of art".

Regarding the bond between one of today's most successful and growing industries and one of the most unsuccessful attempts mankind has ever made and used expanding resources on through an ever more extended time frame I have come to a conclusion in the form of financial statements in permanent imbalance:

- The health industry´s costs are the community´s costs.
- The health industry´s profits are the private owners of the health industry´s profits.

It is difficult for me, impossible, to imagine how these huge players should be able to get into a situation where they have common interests and collaborate. In other words it is equivalently unlikely *that it is from the current treatment regime we expect will give us the solution to the riddle if cancer.*

16. An evaluation of Thoresen´s research

Substances
that our bodies
themselves are producing
that at the first attempt
in the laboratory
shows exactly the qualities
that all cancer researchers
in all the world's
laboratories
have hunted since
the hunt for the solution
of the riddle of cancer
began.

October 2012

After Thoresen had the idea of "translating" the acupuncture method´s effect to biochemistry through laboratory research, so that scientific scholars, doctors and scientists could understand it, he has to my understanding of the scientific evidence actually approached an interesting hypothesis about the solution of the riddle of cancer in principle is about. As described in the chapter about "Chi and chemistry" he and Manzetti has illustrated the process that our body itself produces transmitters that initiates a biochemical defined process that *can* prevent the formation of cancerous tumours, or destroy them, after a temporary defect in the body's growth regulation has allowed the development of symptoms.

According to Thoresen it is in principle simple to complete this research path. His situation will nevertheless be both time consuming and costly to go through the many attempts which have to be implemented, both to be sure about the results but also to expand the research with varying materials (several blood samples from patients with several forms of cancer) for a more accurate overall

231

picture of this part of the organism's "treasure". One will probably get a situation where some things is common, for example for the same type of cancer, but where it also in such cases can be identified individual formation of defence compounds, which can be identified with the types of cancer, and so on.

The "simple" is about being able to get right to the point. One does not need to constantly test new, engineered substances that may inhibit disease symptoms. It is instead a far simpler method; stimulating (with acupuncture), analyse and possibly duplicate what nature has developed through evolution - biological processes throughout our prehistory that has been effective prevention and incapacitation of cancer. What is the secret behind the fact that not everyone gets cancer, and that, thus far, a majority of people is able to keep the defence mechanisms stronger than cancer, is the body's natural ability, from which we find ourselves in the womb, to form the type of cells that can maintain this defence.

Because Thoresen has chosen to give priority to patients and further spread of the method outside Norway[86], I concentrate on this part of his business.

Having immersed myself in the concept of terminal cancer patients and the brutal reality that these people encounter I send an e-mail to Thoresen:

> - *Do you know how many cancer patients you have treated, who have first contacted you after they could no longer be offered treatment in hospitals and therefore were called "terminal"? If so, you may know roughly how many you have been able to help?*

The following circumvention of the questions are promptly returned:

> - The situation for terminal patients involves two serious problems. The most important is the medical assessment of where the line should be drawn that a patient should be described as terminally ill, and when doctors or other

clinicians should inform patients and their families about the likely remaining survival time. The second problem is that doctors or other clinicians who believe the limits are mistakes, has mostly been criminalised. The only thing I will quote about personal experiences with the so-called terminal patients, i.e. those that themselves tell me that they are, is that even those who do not survive, generally live much better after the treatment. I think there should have to be other and stricter criteria to operate with the term terminal. If the criteria really are as you suggest in your question, I will add that I do not see any logical or medical professional justification for using a term terminal on the basis that the patient is no longer offered or recommended continued hospital treatment for the disease.

Two days after I got this answer, 3rd of November 2010[87], and almost as an answer to the question Thoresen had not wanted to answer, was a former featured email, forwarded from Oster Wanner in Switzerland:

Dear Are Thoresen

Three weeks ago E. wrote me, that she is the happiest women in the world because she came to meet your needles. A week later W. told me that his Colon – cancer cannot be found any more & that everybody at the clinic is totally surprised. His neighbour's brain cancer has tremendously reduced in size, and the doctors can't believe what they see. And here in Switzerland, E. feels healthy and does not spent any time thinking about having suffered from cancer.

To sum it up: I did send 4 people to you lately, all of them with severe to infest diagnoses. All 4 are cured or whatever we want to call it.
100 %!
Again!

In the part of the email cited here, O. W. gives a relevant insight to both the treatment method's effectiveness and the question of how dying the so-called terminal patients actually are. Because Thoresen had not wanted to comment specifically about his results with terminal patients, O. W. description of the outcome for the last four Swiss patients who have contacted him for treatment, read as a good and descriptive comment to the question he refused to give a concrete answer to. I can interpolate the reason I asked Thoresen about terminal patients, is that I knew beforehand that it is precisely this group of patients he has the most experience with. For obvious reasons, it is the most severe and final stages of the disease, usually after it has been ascertained metastasis, and/or that treatment is no longer offered, that cancer patients who have heard about his methods and results, also dared to contact him for a very last attempt.

O. W. does not refer many cases - two serious and two terminal - but the result is four of a possible four. Expressed in statistical terms: *100% healed.*

In my first conversation with cancer researcher Mæhlen, shortly after I became acquainted with the email from Oster Wanner, I referred her summary of the four patients' disease progression. His spontaneous comment when I quoted the last part of the email was:

Either this is fraud or the century's medical sensation.

This is mentioned because it is only apparently as simple as Mæhlen portray it. It is of course easy to ascertain whether Thoresen, O. W. and all of us who are trying to spread information about his work, commits fraud or not. It will not take more than a minor effort from an oncologist, preferable from the most sceptical category, which can map Thoresen's treatment of both humans and dogs over a period of time, like Thoresen's own clinical trial, which I will return to below.

However, what has not proved easy so far, is to get someone with medical academic authority to want to carry out such investigation. With the of understanding and experience background

234

that applies to oncologists and cancer researchers at the Norwegian hospitals, where maybe one in a hundred thousand terminal patients and a few per cent of the most severely affected by cancer comes alive through the illness crucial final phase, it is not difficult to imagine that the email from Oster Wanner appears to be a too good news to be true.

It has taken some time to get this script to the finished book. When I'm at the last proofreading I notice that the email from Oster Wanner is no longer recent, I send a request to Thoresen about what became of the four patients from November 2010.

The same day I get the following response by e-mail:

> " Do not know, I do not have the capacity for that kind of follow-up. I almost don't even remember it, I live in the moment with my treatments, possibly that's why I can work at all. But why don't you write to Desi yourself?"

Yes, why not?
Nor O. W. remembered these four patients. The reason is that this is no longer a medical sensation for her.
She answers:

> *"Hi,* Finn.
>
> I did send many more patients to Are. I'll have to check which one you meant and do this tomorrow. I think one is a friend who suffered from colon-CA and the others are probably mamma-CAs. Most people that I sent had conventional treatment as well. Do you want information on them, too, or just on the one or two patients with CA's that had no other treatment? I sent people as soon as they get their diagnosis, and usually they go (to Are – my comment) before they have surgery – thus they usually have their appointments and treatments fixed when they reach Norway and then follow up the routine schedule they did set up in European hospitals when they got diagnosed. This all together works very well,

for the past 10 years I heard only of one person dying – and she seemed to be a lot later starting acupuncture than all the others.

> Come back to you tomorrow.
> Gruss"

I replied that she did not need to dig into what was obviously a much larger patient volume than I had realised, but added that possibly I or others will return to the question later if anyone will examine the history behind what Mæhlen referred to as "the century´s medical sensation".

Ever since he made his discoveries, Thoresen has attempted to share his knowledge with colleagues and professionals in the authorised health care in Norway. So far he has not succeeded in this. A symptomatic approach is an answer he received a few years ago on one of his many inquiries to Norwegian cancer researchers, this time a researcher at the National Hospital, as he had informed about the method and the results he had achieved:

> - This would be too good to be true. Therefore, I don't think it is true.

Though Thoresen has failed to communicate his discoveries at home, however, the knowledge is spread worldwide through an extensive international network of clinicians, veterinarians and doctors who use acupuncture in their practice and have learned to practice the method. It now benefits cancer-sick people in many countries on five continents. I also had contact with clinicians and patients outside Norway, which reinforces the impression Thoresen's own clinical experiences have given me (see appendix).

I have not found any weakness in his own representation of the discovery or the listed references, in short, nothing that could have made me unsure of the clinical study he has conducted and that is presented below.

236

The study's only weakness is that its results have not been confirmed by an independent source. Theoretically, they can therefore be fictional. Now, the purpose of the study was not to provide the final proof of the method's efficacy. It was initiated on the recommendation of one of the Radium hospital´s cancer researchers and therefore something Thoresen had reason to believe was the beginning of a constructive dialogue, perhaps a collaboration with authorised Norwegian Cancer Research. That it was not so, Thoresen says more about below, but it could probably have been the same syndrome (too good results to be believed) which was openly communicated by the researcher from the hospital, namely that after a hundred and fifty years of worldwide cancer research without other than "cosmetic" progress comes a single veterinarian and claims he has cracked the code. It would be "too good to be true".

Thoresen´s work is not considered like this in any country other than Norway. Out in the world he is described as the great master of his discipline, and the method for restoring our natural defences against cancer is held as his masterpiece. Cf. his Irish colleague Roger's description in Chapter 4 ("Who is Are Thoresen?").

In 2012 I got a somewhat special confirmation of Thoresen's reputation abroad, as he that year during an annual convention held at Vienna Veterinary university received a honorary distinction from the Association of Austrian veterinary medicine that uses acupuncture. Moreover, he was the main speaker at the congress.

As the first country Canada has opened the door to a publication of the method and its results in a peer-reviewed journal. After Thoresen lectured about his treatment method in Vancouver at the invitation of the Canadian Association of Medical Acupuncture - an association of doctors who also use acupuncture in their medical work – his treatment method has been discussed in a medical professional *peer review*[88] journal. The author is Michael Greenwood, a doctor who has practiced it for several years[89].

Besides Greenwood an extensive international network of qualified health workers and researchers exists, including at high level of conventional medicine, which currently stands behind my expectation that the treatment method will soon be subject to a critical examination.

oOo

Although I have deferred to comment Thoresen's clinical study, I have suggested that the results are extraordinary. The reason why I have waited to present it is that I paradoxically enough regard it as the greatest obstacle to a constructive dialogue with the Norwegian oncologists and researchers.

From what I've learned about *cancer psychology* I'm sure I would have lost many readers after a few pages if I had started with having to impress them with the results of the study. They are so good that they would create serious scepticism about the author's truthfulness.

Thoresen mentions another example of the effect of presenting the study in the academic community:

> - When I had treated so many that I was quite sure of the method's effect, and wanted to publish it, I understood the need to first complete a form of statistics. I know little about the formal requirements for publication of research results. Therefore, I contacted a researcher who then worked at the Norwegian Radium Hospital. In the conversations I was careful to anticipate any result. As long as I asked for advice on how I should conduct a clinical examination, I received very good help. Two years later when I sent the researcher the outcome of the study, I got no answer. Repeated messages via voice mail, email, and other people in the same department gave no response.
> - *This sounds strange - that a qualified researcher, who must be assumed to have normal general politeness, closes for communication in such a way?*
> - Yes, I know it may sound strange, but this is far from the only time constructive conversations and plans have suddenly stopped and been replaced by silence.

- Have you thought about what could be your share of the responsibility for this to have happened?
- To be honest, this has been such great disappointment that I have not had the energy for anything other than managing my own reactions. When it was done, I again concentrated on my work instead of analysing why others stop answering the phone.
- But you've still made some thoughts?
- Of course, but I say as the former Justice Minister Storberget when a journalist from NRK asked about his views on an unkind statement from the Iranian embassy: "I have made some thoughts, but keep them to myself."

On the other hand, Thoresen can give examples of doctors within the authorised research community that has helped him to convey his results: In the spring of 2010, he wanted to publish an article based on a newly developed form of acupuncture treatment of horses with equine sarcoid (one type of skin cancer in horses with no known healing treatment). He got help with the design of the text of a physician with research as his daily work, namely Fønnebø at Tromsø Hospital (and as earlier mentioned head of NAFKAM). The article was sent to the *Equine Veterinary Education*, one of the world's most recognised magazines in terms of disease in horses. Basis of the article was the treatment of 18 sick horses.

This may be referred to as a minor clinical trial. The result of this is that the treatment was ineffective on two horses. The remaining 16 recovered completely as in the tumours shrank and disappeared, all within a period of six weeks. On two of the horses that recovered, tumours came back after two years. Repeated treatment removed the tumours again.

While he was helped to write the article by Fønnebø, the response from the editors was negative. The rejection was entirely justified by formal errors. The only comment to the survey was why Thoresen had only used 18 horses and not a number that would have provided a better statistical basis.

The answer reveals how little reality oriented such consultants may be. The study includes namely all cases of the disease Thoresen has come into contact with as far back as 1995, i.e. a period of fifteen years.

As he himself put it: "If it had been possible to gather a hundred horses with the disease, the result would probably be similar".

Even an amateur (non-consultant in a scientific journal) will understand that healing 16 out of 18 horses for a nearly un-curable disease does not happen by accident. The concrete result, the core of the article, a result that I know no one else has come close to achieving, was not mentioned with a word. I ask myself why the editors are not curious enough that they take up the main theme in their feedback to the author.

A positive factor in connection with the article on equine sarcoids was the help Thoresen received from Fønnebø. When I heard about this constructive dialogue, I suggested that he could send Fønnebø the mail he had received from Oster Wanner from Switzerland (regarding the two severe and two terminal cancer patients who had all become healthy). There was immediate answer from Fønnebø:

> *- This seems to be very interesting stories. We would love to have them in our register of exceptional courses of disease.*

This is positive feedback, but at the same time I am a little disappointed that this does not lead to a more proactive attitude to want to verify whether Thoresen really can achieve 100% healing in disease conditions where the cancer wards in all of Western Hospital has a statistic down to a few% (severe diagnosis) or 0% (terminal diagnosis).

Among the few positive feedbacks on Thoresen's research from the academic community in Norway, it is ultimately one I particularly want to highlight. After I got "a foot inside" at the Norwegian Radium Hospital, the then retiring director of the hospital,

Jan Vincent Johannessen, became so interested of what I passed of my own experiences with the treatment method that he asked Steinar Aamdal to put those researchers who are most experienced with this type of laboratory research to review and assess Manzetti´s research results.

Among stack of medical records and other documentation at my disposal, is a document with Aamdal´s signature, where the following subordinate clause summarises the results of the review of Manzetti´s material carried by the two foremost researchers on Aamdal´s department (according to himself):

To date unknown peptides have in laboratory experiments demonstrated that they neutralise aggressive breast cancer cells.

Although Aamdal´s conclusion on the hospital's review of the laboratory tests and the request to execute multiple (and very expensive) laboratory experiments was a kind of a "good day, man axe handle" response to my request for a collaboration on the discovery, this subordinate clause may prove to be almost as important as Aamdal had directly agreed to such cooperation. Instead he conducted himself to my questions that I virtually ruled over unlimited resources for cancer research and therefore come back when this was explored in the same degree as when a drug manufacturer addressed to him regarding the testing of a new cancer drug.

Clinical research (testing on humans) constitute a significant source of revenue for the Norwegian Radium Hospital, which is paid by the pharmaceutical industry. Should the Radium Hospital further research Thoresen´s hypotheses and preliminary results, other and higher authorities within the health care system than Aamdal himself may decide it. Here is possibly the explanation for his refusal and regardless a great challenge.

In this context it is important to emphasise that help to further exploration and testing should be considered from commercial goals and interests. Thoresen´s discovery and basic research, according to his statement and documented arrangements is his contribution to the community, notably if the research is carried on their own terms so that it is neither absorbed by commercial interests or parked like a defeated contender for the chemical industry.

oOo

As mentioned, I am initially sceptical about the usefulness of patient stories if they are not included in a documentable relationship or is so thoroughly documented as the "patient diary" that is the basis of this book. However, I had noted the exceptional results with the four Swiss patients (see E-mail from Oster Wanner) and also wanted to establish contact with some of Thoresen´s Norwegian patients.

In my view, he has a somewhat excessive ethical approach to his work, which meant that I initially did not get on with my work. His attitude and response to my request was that he believes it is wrong of him to ask some of the patients to share their experiences with the treatment. I have wondered about this, and given that this was early in our relationship about the book (November 2010) the first thought was, naturally enough, that there could be a hidden motive, something he actually wanted to hide. This occupied me so much that it also ended with me a few days later got an idea of how I could get around this ethical roadblock.

I asked if I could be allowed to hang up a poster in his waiting room that briefly described the book project, and that I wanted to get in contact with patients who has cancer or had cancer and felt they had something important to tell me. He agreed that it was an acceptable solution, and after a few days I asked him to take down the poster again. Enough patients to confirm the impression I had formed had called me, and that it would not be problematic to find Norwegian patients who could share their experiences with the treatment they have received if others want to make a similar evaluation.

Of those who called were two who had witnessed aggressive cancer that so far is termed as incurable, like squamous cell carcinoma in dogs[90] and equine sarcoma in horses were healed in a

242

short time, usually 5-6 weeks after treatment by Thoresen and without recurrence. I also talked with patients who have gone through something similar to what I have experienced, though not as the sole treatment.

In addition to she who tells her story online (note 87) I refer from the conversation with a well-grown man who was struck by leukaemia. He was one of the few with serious cancer that had sought Thoresen early, and he received an acupuncture treatment before he started chemotherapy. The doctors had told him that the high dose chemotherapy that was necessary in his case, probably would be especially demanding. Loss of appetite, nausea, weight loss, fatigue, gloom, hair loss and impaired immune system was side effects he was prepared to be hit with. I recognised these side effects from other patients' descriptions that had undergone normal and far less stressful chemotherapy. "Felleskatalogen" (the Norwegian PDR) confirms this and also lists several other, more dangerous side effects, which affects smaller percentages of patients.

The leukaemia patient noticed no side effects whatsoever. Every day he went for long walks with his dog. He had a good appetite and heard underway in the treatment from the doctors that his immune system was in such good condition that they could not understand how that was possible.

Furthermore, the patient could tell that at no time after Thoresen´s treatment samples were taken which indicated that he still had cancer. To me he seemed completely unconcerned, without fear of recurrence. He was full of gratitude that he was one of the few who had the opportunity to receive this treatment.

A main principle for a clinical study is that all patients will be enrolled in the study. I have asked Thoresen to undergo the raw material for the article where he presents the results of his treatment. He has never had a secretary. Therefore, the background information could have been better and more systematically filed. Most patients have indeed survived the disease(!) and will thus be able to participate in a thorough evaluation of the study. Yet I would suggest the use of resources in a new study, where independent professionals take care of both secretarial work and the final conclusions.

Based on the material I have available, I made my own summary of the method's results. This was primarily intended to satisfy my own curiosity to get an indication of how effective the treatment is. I had previously immersed myself thoroughly in cancer statistics, and also decided in this case to create my own statistics. The first thing I did was to *grade the different cases from a set of criteria I had previously set up*.

> • If the tumour has diminished or disappeared when other strategies than those offered on the cancer wards, this has until now been regarded as a special medical exception or an impossibility, and has been characterised as anecdotal healing. For these cases, I use the term *unusually great effect*.
> • If the growth of cancer tumours have stopped after acupuncture treatment, this means in most cases healing. It is the treatment that halts growth, not any subsequent removal by surgery, which is the cause of healing. For such cases, I use the term *lasting effect*.
> • If growth has stopped or the tumour has shrunk or disappeared altogether, but it has begun to grow again or come back at a later date, it is about healing with relapse. This could just as easily be due to external circumstances or the patient's lifestyle that is deficient in the treatment - here termed *effect with relapse*.
> • The tumour continues to grow as untreated tumours normally do, indicating that the treatment has had *no effect*.

I will then received the following categories:

> • Exceptionally great effect
> • Lasting effect
> • Effect with relapse
> • No effect

In Thoresen's study patients are followed over such a short period of time that one can not know enough about any recurrence in the first two categories. It is also in my view other inadequately mapped parameters. Particularly lacking in each case a thorough investigation of the extent to which hospital treatment has been able to influence the outcome.

However, what interests us here is *whether the trial at all confirms that the treatment has a significant effect* - something that it in my view does. Then possibly a new, supervised experiment where Thoresen will receive help with the formal and technical aspects, enhancing the study's degree of precision.

I have in Chapter 13 ("Is it presented evidence for Thoresen's treatment method") referenced a type of *qualitative study*, that is, with only one person. The example is based on my patient diary and its documentation, the hospital record. After I got acupuncture treatment, the cancer became better, contrary to all prognoses for this disease's normal development. Later, when the disease recurred twice during the first eighteen months after diagnosis, the disease disappeared again immediately after the new targeted acupuncture treatment. In one case the treatment strategy was also changed. Thoresen's own assessment was that both the tangible and measurable growth of the tumour was due to a lack of control of his part. In the second case, growth was much faster, and also led to a very dramatic situation the oncologist describes in the medical record as "likely inoperable" and in this case also incurable. In all three cases, after diagnosis and two subsequent relapses, did the effect of the treatment show so rapidly that it was detected at the early controls by MRI and in the first case also by biopsies. In the diary from this time I write:

> "If my plea for a minor surgical procedure without prior
> radiation had been heard, I would after the regrowth of the
> tumour which came after the Avastin treatment, chosen to
> get the tumour removed, since such an operation would

result in much less risk of permanent damage than the traditional and more extensive cancer surgery. For me there was no longer any doubt about the acupuncture treatment´s level of precision, which was abundantly confirmed by the hospital's most precise measuring tools, PET CT.

To stress the tumour once more with cancer hazardous radiation and cut away as much as possible to catch any cancer cells "hiding in corners outside the tumour", as one surgeon put it, was something I thought was unnecessary vandalism on my body. Moreover, it was based on an opposite approach to cancer than the treatment I had chosen."

As an example of my assessment of the individual cases in Thoresen´s clinical trial may I add that if I had been one of the participants, I would, regardless of the treatment´s quality, had to be placed in the second worst of the four categories mentioned above, namely the effect with recurrence, possibly with a note that two relapses had known causes, and that they probably had not occurred if these reasons had been absent.

The benefit with dogs in the study is that in this case the uncertainty if it is the acupuncture treatment or authorised medications that cause the effect is absent. I would add that if what I have learned about the effects of hospital treatment in the cases of cancer that are represented in the study, I consider this uncertainty as small even for people. While Thoresen has succeeded to treat aggressive breast cancer that has spread, we know from the statistics that the probability that the same disease will continue to diminish after hospital treatment with chemotherapy, radiation and surgery are very small. The reason that most patients would seek other treatment, was precisely that the disease had worsened after hospital treatment, and that both hope of survival and the statistical chances of survival has become even smaller. In other words, hospital treatment do not seem to have any significant impact on the number of healings or the number of patients registered with the effect of the treatment.

The way I've structured the summary of Thoresen´s results, is due to considerations of both readability and the need to review the material from scratch, which however has been shown to have little impact on the final result. Because I've done it this way, I have references Thoresen's own description in the appendix.

The overview includes all of Thoresen´s patients with cancer through eighteen months. Overall, it involves 34 patients, where it is reported back results from 28, which breaks down as 12 people and 16 animals (15 dogs and one horse). I've only interacted with the results from these 28 patients. The last six have either not been back for further treatments or not given feedback on the development.

That six of the original 34 patients dropped out would have been a problem if the experiment had been the basis for a scientific study. Therefore this must be read as a summary of the available material, as an indication and far from any evidence - an indication that the procedure should be further studied and undergo a real scientific study[91].

The results I have as best placed within the categories mentioned above.

	Animals(An)	People(P)	All(A)	An%	P%	A%
Exceptionally effect	7	5	12	44	42	43
Lasting effect	5	6	11	31	50	40
Effect with relapse	3	1	4	19	8	14
No effect	1	0	1	6	0	3
Total effect	16	12	28	94	100	97

Although the study did not include more than 28 participants, it seems obvious, at least to me, that the method has so much effect on cancers that it should be a treatment option for anyone who wants it. Then I assume of course that the results are repeated in controlled studies. If I in some cases may have placed the patient in the wrong group, it is not possible to make mistakes when it comes to patients in the last group. One dog showed no improvement is apparently that only one of both animals and humans where it was not noted effect of the treatment.

An effect of 97% is a lot, so much that no cancer researchers so far have shown confidence that the results are based on actual conditions. What will now be new compared to how Thoresen have presented his research on acupuncture before, is that these results can be considered in the context of the laboratory research of Manzetti and the conclusion I got from the Norwegian Radium Hospital after their review of the laboratory experiments. When Steinar Aamdal has confirmed that scientists at his department has found that the peptides that the body has produced minutes after a cancer patient has received acupuncture treatment has shown efficacy in cancer cells in the laboratory, I understand this as a clear, though indirect, confirmation of the acupuncture´s effect on the immune system.

It is thirty years since Thoresen in his first attempt to test the method healed a dog with advanced cancer. During this time he has treated more than 600 Norwegian cancer cases (humans, dogs and horses). The efforts familiarise myself with what has happened in those years, and the attempt to convey it has engaged me so strongly that I sometimes fear that it will be a new thirty years before people with cancer get offered this treatment.

Whenever fear comes, however, it quickly is replaced by renewed optimism and excitement related to who I meet around the next corner, and who have something constructive to contribute. That several cancer researchers are interested in talking to me, has already been a positive surprise.

oOo

When I tell my friends and associates what I'm dealing with, I get with slight variations the same reaction:

- But this is amazing!

In spontaneous credulity they take for granted that this will soon benefit those with cancer. Credulity is because they do not have experienced how powerful economic interests that prevail within a sector of society most people take for granted is both academically independent and governed by humanitarian considerations.

The desire to get rich and richer, is natural to man. In everyday life he is himself closest either in terms of economy, power or glory. That a single veterinarian comes with the "solution" and a type of solution that puts most of the on-going cancer research and treatment in the shade, do not awaken spontaneously professional enthusiasm and is neither spreading like wildfire in the medical research communities.

That I still look favourably on the possibility that Thoresen´s method can be implemented in a relatively close future, is mainly due to that I believe information and knowledge about it will spread and lead to a collective requirement that the treatment is made available to more Norwegians than now, via random information, find their way to the small one-man clinic in Sandefjord.

It is the patients and their spokesmen and women, the independent general practitioners and especially journalists and politicians who may be fire in the dry grass as they, as I think and hope, demands from the medical elite that patients interests come first.

17. A community perspective

Although treatment methods have been improved and perfected in line with technological advances, cancer has still not become any less of a problem for people. Statistics on the number of cancer deaths in the last fifty years is steadily rising[92]. If we compare these statistics with the Cancer Registry statistics for the number of diagnoses, we could predict that in a relatively short time, from a historical perspective, there will be

- a higher number of Norwegians which receive a cancer diagnosis than those who will not, and that
- about a quarter of the population will have cancer as cause of death

if a radical change does not occur within an even shorter time in the understanding and treatment of cancer diseases.

When it comes to the profession that has the most closely contact with cancer patients, i.e. nurses, I can tell that I have not met a single one who has expressed nothing but joy and optimism when I have told about what has cured my disease. Nobody in this category of health workers objected to the fact that I waited to be operated on to see if the cure was permanent. Nine out of ten doctors working in cancer wards, however, had a clear negative attitude towards my choices. I imagine that those same doctors will smile of the nurses' naivety and gullibility, while the *one* (out of ten) will appreciate their openness and good faith. However, I understand that the doctors 'role is to be sceptical of anything that might be a threat to patients' health or their own professional integrity, and see this as an understandable and respectable position if they could show the same respect and understanding for the patients who take responsibility for their own health and make independent choices.

Among GPs, I have the impression that there are far more that are both frustrated with the situation and open to new and less harmful treatments *if only the effect can be documented in a satisfactory manner*. One of them, Ragnar Sundby, who runs a small clinic in Vestfold, says he does not know a single GP in his local community he thinks would have qualms that cancer patients receive acupuncture treatment if it can be shown that it can actually help them. If he is right, there is hope of specific changes both in the attitude to cancer diseases and their treatment, and also that these can happen fairly quickly.

To achieve a reduction in the steadily rising incidence of cancer, there is not treatment, but only preventive efforts that have effect.

250

Though I have devoted great space for the vitamin D´s significance it must not be understood that there are no other vitamins or supplements that are important for protection against cancer. I would therefore reiterate that approximately 10,000 studies that have found associations between cancer and diet have been conducted, based on the quality and quantity of the food and beverages we put in our body. In the literature on this it is claimed to have solid evidence that there is a lot every cancer patient should know about nutrition physiology and pay attention to their way of life. When this research has not led to cancer, physicians generally have a more active approach to how patients live and eat, it must be because it is in this environment a strong belief that diet has no decisive effect for the further course of the disease.

How has this prejudice occurred? Because I have so far only seen research that argues the opposite, I have concluded that the aforementioned dogma that *only authorised cancer treatment can reverse the course of cancer*, along with *a very successful marketing of this dogma* must have a stronger influence than 10,000 studies showing that the opposite is the case, even within a professional group which particularly emphasises that it is only natural science research results of high quality that counts. I would think that none of those who govern our cancer care believes that the 10,000 studies it refers to are of too poor quality to be considered.

At this point I get an outrageous thought, which should be an obvious fact also for everyone else if they only allow such a huge outrage to penetrate the shell of innocence that protects us from asking about what we cannot do anything about.

If I had not with an increasing clarity realised how bad it can be when medical research is at the mercy of investors and the financial sector's cynicism, I had not referred it:

Patients' health is the health industry's biggest competitor.

There is no way out of this impasse. It is difficult if not impossible to imagine that a form of finance-Darwinism or worldwide practice with a monopolised market and the players need to enrich themselves could give us a "healthy" health care system. The only solution is, as I see it, a form of production of drugs in which all parties and participants have common interests.

This has nothing to do with a critique of capitalism or a stand for right-or left-wing politics. It's as simple as that *when the almost death of one is the other's bread*, they constitute together a constellation in which both parties in the long run is in conflict with themselves and kill their own fruits. For pharmaceutical manufacturers the market capitalism is no real growth factor, but an arena where it happens all too much play and pointless innovation on other community sector's expense. Therefore this analysis concludes that there is not in all circumstances, and especially not in this, that capitalism and market forces (even if they were free and not monopolistic) is expedient life. Mankind will certainly not be healthier in this system, where it is needed a former super capitalists like Bill Gates and his 100bn for an attempt to allocate the right medications (and vaccines) in a fair way in the world. Cancer development in the West are too much to take on even for the American billionaire, despite the fact that he is said to have been joined by more than a hundred other billionaires on his project.

In my thoughts on how this situation can be reversed, I urged my mind's eye into a far from distant past where the apothecary mixed his potions solely on what he thought was best for the patients. This was a time when it was out of the question to imagine that other motives played in, and where, for example, it was not mixed unnecessary substances that were addictive so one could increase revenue[93]. General ethics said that this was absurd: it would change the medication to something close to the opposite of medicine. I looked back at a time when ethics and economics within the local medicine production went hand in hand without anyone else ever questioned it. That is just how it was. The goal of the apothecary was

252

patient safety rather than earning more money by having other more important tasks facing those who owned the pharmacy.

In the future, I envision a situation with only common interests between patients and pharmaceutical manufacturers. I believe this can be achieved if Norway or other Scandinavian countries continue governing the modernisation and technification of its health care system. None of the players will be able to have a desire for continued growth in the healthcare industry. On the contrary. If the state assumes responsibility for the development and production of drugs, the overall design is to develop drugs that make people healthier. It will also focus on medication that makes itself superfluous, than drugs that make patients into long-term users of drugs, as is the case with a large proportion of the medicines we import. For cancer diseases statistics prove that this has been the trend over the past fifty years. Although the statistics called "Survival"[94] is meant to hide the fact that there are no more Norwegian cancer patients that survive today than it was fifty years ago, these statistics document, certainly involuntary, that the increasing number of people every year who get the disease, becomes dependent on medical and health service in a continually extended period of time. The consequence is that the state and the patients have to pay larger and larger sums for medications, which in turn causes increased social security payments. Economically regarded both preventive measures, such as regular monitoring of the population's vitamin D supply, and the introduction of natural curative cancer treatment, as this book testifies is developed in Norway and on a small scale in use worldwide with overwhelmingly positive results, provide benefits for all with the exception of a few speculators and some small investors who are incapable of understanding what they have helped to finance.

If we continue as at present, with the rapid growth in the number of cancer cases and generally zero growth in the number of survivors, it will result in a loss for all but a few investors and individual equity savers if they do not get cancer and have to taste their own medicine.

oOo

A lot of vital and useful chemical medicine is produced, but the chemical industry markets and sells large quantities of useless and even harmful products.

At one time also Thoresen had ambition to produce a chemically manufactured medicine, but in a different and new "division". Instead of *symptom suppressors* it was talk of *disease removers* based on the model of the "medicines" our organism itself creates.

I have the impression that this ambition is now abandoned. In the book, I have argued that Manzetti´s laboratory research, which admittedly is a first step towards such a medicine, has already proven that Thoresen´s acupuncture treatment strengthens the immune system against cancer. The same mechanism that apply for this treatment form, may according to Thoresen and Manzetti´s research also apply to many health problems and illnesses where acupuncture is effective. This is how Thoresen/Manzetti has opened for an extended research on the changes in the blood that occurs immediately after a successful treatment against in principle all conditions where acupuncture has shown clinical efficacy[95]. In my view this is a far more important goal to reach than having to produce a chemical copy, which is then patented and put into production in the same way as today's chemical medications.

The bridges built between acupuncture and natural sciences already completed, is "just"[96] missing an objective scientific documentation so that other researchers can build on this platform - towards a global medicine which is also inclusive because it does not have to compete with other medications. This medication will not be patentable, and therefore will not be a speculative object for investors.

oOo

Although all professions are more or less important to ensure a qualitatively good society, it is my contention that health care as a whole is in a unique position. It is natural to compare them with those

254

professions that enhance our life situation through enforcement of our laws, and ensure us against abuse of any kind from various individual stakeholders or interest groups.

In my view, an effort should be made to end the remnant of ancestral hierarchy and "guild protection", which in the health care system can provide greater negative and dramatic effect than in most other occupational groups[97]. This forerunner of the modern-day unions of alternative practitioners have dated back to the "wise women´s" time and have been excluded. This has probably contributed to that they, for generations, have been left at the bottom of the hierarchy as a large common category. Regardless of their knowledge and qualifications they are put in the "same box" and they are not heard within the decision-making process in a way that is reasonable in relation to their actual positions in the Health Care in Norway - measured by the number of treatments and the results thereof, as evaluated by their patients.

A requirement often made by public authorities to alternative practitioners is that they should not have as a motive to make money. If they do not meet the expectation of a high degree of idealism and economic austerity, it can alone lead to suspicion about both the lack of integrity and professional incompetence.

At the same time there is great indulgence with the fact that virtually all government-approved drugs are produced with a single motive for the greatest possible financial profit for the companies who make them. Here I again associate to "marketing effect", i.e. the type of marketing that affect us without our knowing. This phenomenon is discussed in Chapter 15 ("Ethics and Economics in cancer treatment"), but with the difference that it concerns an indirect and "negative" form of marketing. It is usually no longer appropriate to promote your own project by disparaging descriptions of competitors. In the health sector, this happens in a way that will make the "market" believe that it's not about competition for patients, but communication of realities - shelter by the knowledge that is awarded the academic recognised and classified categories of skilled health workers. An example of this indirect and often aggressive promotion

255

is the claim that alternative practitioners' "shoes themselves on the cancer patients' expense" - an accusation which targets at random, as all are treated "with the same brush". The accusation is all the more gross and unfair as the small practitioner is set up against some of the richest in the world, a handful of major shareholders in the cancer industry, which are those we rightly should have addressed this accusation against.

I have tried to show that the economy motif results in numerous and often costly medications we do not need, and that can be harmful or directly dangerous and that we miss a plethora of good and helpful medications from smaller and less financially strong competitors. What I will present as a hopefully effective "emergency medicine" against this policy is that the government takes over the "economy motif". One should then begin with an evaluation of the affordable and almost free preventive and curative strategies against cancer that is described in the book, while undertake an evaluation of current money-drain strategies. Both should be based on accurate statistics and objective scientific studies.

The evaluation may lead to a reduction of costs associated with cancer treatment and corresponding increased efforts on a number of other health areas where we know we are getting results for every dollar invested. Likewise it may show that we through decades has spent a fortune on import of anticancer drugs without significant effect.

Although I for my part initially was aware that a lot of the drug production took place at private production facilities, I thought, however, that the public sector's role in the development of new drugs was larger than it is. In reality, the public has no or minimal control of the development and manufacturing of medications we are offered, nor with their costs and prices. The government's power is limited to accept or reject, while a significant portion of the western states' health budgets disappear in the international financial sector.

Life is about building expectations and illusions and then lose them again. I lost many of those I had about our modern, western health care while working on this book.

In such a situation it is easy to be unilateral and transmit the lost illusions of a "system" at all occupational groups - professionals and bureaucrats - and everything they do. It can be hard not to get carried away in disillusionment´s downward spiral, where the bottom may end with an easily acquired embellishment of opposites to the idols that failed.

An example from my side to try to keep *judgment* (not necessarily objectivity) is that I have not wanted to refute the key arguments that strongly justifies protectionism of the pharmaceutical industry, who really is not about protecting the pharmaceutical industry, but to protect patients against unscientific treatment. This argument I could not agree more with.

I so agree that *I profoundly disagree that there are not requirements for all health professionals*, but only to those who are associated with the authorised treatment forms. The alternative health care is about the only group without requirements from society, in spite of the exceptionally important and responsible task they take on by opening a clinical practice.

One effect of this is, whether it is intentional or not, is that the entire group of alternative health workers are treated as if they are poorly academically qualified to treat serious diseases such as cancer. On the contrary, it should be requirement for them that they can reasonably fulfil, requirements include evidence of their competence, whether they have a degree or invoke special powers that make education redundant, so that they too can offer assistance to cancer patients at the level that their expertise dictates. The assistance may include the full spectrum of counselling on nutrition, lifestyle, attitudes, thoughts and feelings to involve clinicians with both broad and deep medical background, but who lack formal medical qualifications. As mentioned, the new law on alternative therapies in 2003 is a step in the right direction, but it is necessary to proceed in the same direction.

By having requirements to all health care professionals and providing authorisations at the different levels and documentation requirements adapted to the various qualifications, both the protectionism of the pharmaceutical industry and "guild protection" within the health care system is weakened and perhaps even finally broken.

A prime example of what effects "guild protection" of the authorised health care provides, is the fact that on average more than ten people die at Norwegian hospitals due to improper treatment and that more than five patients per day die as a result of errors solely caused by hospital personnel.

If hospital patients had been airplanes and not people, not one of those serious mistakes would be tolerated without consequences for the person, work situation or the "system" that was responsible for the error.

The terrible death statistics from 2011 is surprising and almost incredible that I had not dared to refer to them if I had not heard the then Health Minister, Anne Grete Strøm-Erichsen, referring to them on the evening news in September 2012. One can easily imagine the dramatic consequences including media coverage and legal actions that would happen if a clinician who was not doctor- or hospital guild protected, demonstrably wrongly treated one of his patients with death as the result.

The point here is not to criticise, the health minister herself ensured that, but to prove discrimination in favour of certain occupational groups and to the disadvantage of those who will live with or will die from the consequences of unequal treatment. Patients will most obvious benefit that it is not only opened to free competition in the drug market, but also on the market for different treatment methods, and especially with regard to the quality of the methods that are being practiced. Facing similar criticism has defenders of the existing system previously pointed out that the error rate is not large compared with the number of treated patients, which to my ears sounds as absurd as if the technicians in charge of a casualty should invoke the number of successful completed flights.

oOo

None of the criticisms that are put forth in the book is written from a romantic dream of the past or to polarise the current contradictions between authorised and alternative health care. The aim is to find out where we stand today and what opportunities we have to improve the situation, which is easily expressed by that more than the approximately 11,000 Norwegians who died of the disease in 2011, will suffer the same fate year after year.

Assuming that at some point an objective examination of Thoresen's method to treat patients with severe cancer is carried out - with the metastasis and statistically low probability of survival - there must be asked a crucial question:

What percentage of healing beyond the normal statistical norm must the method demonstrate in order to be offered to cancer patients at Norwegian hospitals?

If the method only helps 1% of the patients, it will be a failure in relation to expectations Thoresen's own clinical study has created among us who think it gives a reasonably correct expression for the method's effectiveness. Nevertheless, it would then, given that it was offered to all cancer patients characterised as *inoperable*[98] or terminal, *save a Norwegian life every third day*!

10% would also be a poor outcome compared with our expectations, but the method will result in *three lifesaving treatments a day*!

At an acceptable result it will, in my view, in most cases, be appropriate to use the method as a supplement to existing cancer treatments. In some cases, such as mine, it may turn out that the patient does not need other treatment. It could in fact be situations that quickly changes the patients' diagnosis of cancer diseased to healthy, something my patient diary and medical history is an example of. What happened in my case was that acupuncture treatment, which began the very next day after I got diagnosed with cancer, removed the key symptom (active cancer cells in the tumour) so rapidly that it also removed the established criteria to start authorised cancer treatment.

Assuming that this did not happen as the result of chance, which statistical calculations in general shows may not be the case (see Chapter 9: "About the laboratory research"), the acupuncture treatment will, *because according Thoresen in the majority of cases it has shown a very rapid response*, probably eliminate intensive hospital treatment for a high number of patients the method has an effect on[99]. The weeks it normally takes from diagnosis to an eventual treatment with chemotherapy, radiation or surgery, is in many cases sufficient to establish whether acupuncture has the expected and decisive effect or not. It is at this point - control the effect by biopsy, CT and MRI - that the interaction between traditional Eastern and modern Western methods are essential. Although acupuncturists who practice pulse diagnosis, can to a greater or lesser extent read if the treatment is having the desired effect, this control is by no means as reliable in terms of the precise changes in disease progression pathologists, radiologists and oncologists can read using the hospital's technological equipment and determine through its own expertise in cancer.

In the cases where post-test indicates that acupuncture does not work, this means no lost time relative to the initiation of other treatments. As shown by particularly one patient example in Chapter 16 ("An evaluating of Thoresen´s research") it may in such cases be given complementary acupuncture treatment that reduces the side effects of authorised treatment. Such treatment is given in many western hospitals, including the Hospital of Vestfold, where a considerable amount of research has been conducted in this area[100]. General palliative care, especially if the patient's internal organs like the liver and kidneys are weakened by prolonged medication, old age or other causes, is also a valuable help for the patient, although Thoresen´s method has not successfully cured him of the disease.

oOo

So far, acupuncture has in the book been treated as an Eastern medical tradition. It is both right and wrong. The discovery of a five thousand year old man hiking in the Alps a few years ago is a sure indication that acupuncture in the distant past was not limited to Asia, but was also prevalent in Europe. In all probability, the man was the first ever identified doctor because he had acupuncture needles in his travel bag and tattooed on the body a "map" showing acupuncture meridians and the most commonly used acupuncture points. In many populous cultures, acupuncture is still the most common healing method. Something that is little known, even in Norway, the Sami have traditionally had a private acupuncture system with more than 100 registered points.

Today acupuncture is used in varying degrees in rich and poor countries, yet within a common horizon of understanding. The consequence of this is that a new acupuncture method that is proven somewhere soon may be known and practiced all over the globe.

In the appendix, it is cites a number of specific examples of how Thoresen's treatment against cancer today is disseminated in a global context. Here I include the last three feedbacks he has received from his patients on their own initiative. Two of them have also been able to provide detailed documentation. One of the feedbacks is from Costa Rica (12/24/13), the other from Switzerland (01/04/14). The third and last, which applies to a dog with leukaemia, is from Norway (29/01/14). This is the most interesting in the scientific sense because of the type of documentation. From the School of Veterinary Science in Oslo, through the dog's owner, Thoresen has been given a description on the condition of the dog along with diagrams from blood samples before and after treatment, and a thorough description from a representative of the owner, a Norwegian security company. E-mail sent by the owner of the dog Mighty is shown on the last page of the appendix. Other documentations are in my archive.

One thing is hopefully to have demonstrated the potential health, economic, and overall charitable aspects that the new knowledge about the importance of vitamin D and Thoresen's curative treatment may have for our country and far beyond all borders. Unfortunately, this knowledge has not previously reached the academic community in Norway, partly due to too little and too poor scientific documentation produced.

I also discovered for me novel negative aspects of our health care system, but choose in this summary to appeal to the best aspects of health care to use the presented knowledge in the best way. As in seeking more and deeper knowledge and process it in a way only the authorised health care system can do so it can both be beneficial to as many cancer patients as possible and reverse the trend of increasing the percentage of cancer patients to a situation where the statistics finally can show that a prevention really works.

What can be conveyed already now is in the closing of the book to strengthen the hope that the knowledge and expertise that lies potent underneath the documentation's surface – and in the rest of the material I have introduced – will not be continued to be exported because the Norwegian health care system will not accept the invitation to examine this closer.

18. Epilogue
From political highest level

It was never intended that this book should have the character of a documentary, except from the interviews with the two key researchers and the introductory text from "patient diary".

The events that have taken place after the text was finished in 2013, and until the new proofreading of the content and final editing in February 2014, however, is so suspenseful and relevant that I chose to end the book with an epilogue in diary form, as they unfolded and a minimum of interference from my side.

June 2013
The manuscript was finished, it was good weather and some of them I appreciate being with, went down to the fjord. What I thought was

the beginning of the holiday was instead the beginning of a series of events I had to address before I sent the script. I did not even have time to dip my toes in the water before I got a concerned message from Thoresen where he asked if he could disturb me with a phone call. He could, and when I heard what it was about, it was a short walk back to the desk and a strange e-mail he sent me about the intervention from the "highest political level". The intervention applied to what has for a time had been scheduled to be the first scientific evidence of the effects of his cancer treatment in dogs. This is not mentioned in the book because Thoresen previously would not have any awareness of the experiment because, as he said:

> - This is the third time I've prepared myself to be able to provide scientific evidence for the efficacy of my treatment method. As you know, the first two were stopped without explanation and without my even have been meeting those who vetoed.

Yes, I knew everything about thirty years of struggle at home to have the opportunity to put forward his claims about the method's clinical results. To pay for such an attempt that was now embarked, would cost millions. That a student, Margit Buen at Telemark University College had chosen such an attempt as her thesis, was really an opportunity to finally present the method and its effect in the journals where it could get its deserved attention.

> - Now it's already leaked to the wrong recipient, so now you can write what you want about the experiment,

was his first comment to the e-mail he had received from Buen and forwarded to me. We agreed to talk again when I read it.

I put the cell phone in my pocket, the wet toes in my shoes and left the shore. If I had been a bit annoyed by the curtailment of the summer's first beach visit, such feelings became subordinates the ones I got as I read the email. It was from the editor of the membership magazine of the Norwegian Kennel Klub (NKK), Dog Sports, and the club's Facebook pages, Stepanka Horakova:

- I have now been told by politicians at the highest level that we cannot front the project, and that the case must be removed from our website. Sorry, but I cannot get anything done about this.

The message is forwarded Thoresen from Buen with the following comment:

- Well. I have returned a question of "who politically highest level" is. Expecting a good response. How is it possible!

Buen has a background as a nurse, but also practice natural medicine, psychotherapy and horsemanship[103]. She is in the process of completing her academic education at Telemark University College (HIT). To obtain a sufficient number of dogs, in all sixty-four, for the procedure to reach statistical significance and scientific importance, Buen and HIT was offered help in recruiting cancer dogs by NKK.

Our display e-mail precedes a tail of correspondence with NKK. Previously she has written (May 13):

"I have now got the approval of my project from FDU [The Norwegian Animal Research Authority, my remark]. This trial is the first of its kind and may be important in efforts to develop treatments in tackling cancer. I hope you can post a notice in the Dog Sports about the trial."

Someone who signs by Espen answers:

"I will forward your mail to the editor of Dog Sports, which makes all decisions about what is included in the magazine.

Communications manager/editor Horakova then confirm through the rest of the emails that NKK will work with Buen/HIT on recruitment of dogs, and that the cooperation will include publication in Dog Sports, alternatively NKKs website and Facebook page if it becomes too late to do it in the next issue of the magazine.

It will be interesting, I thought, to see who has rejected a Norwegian university and Animal Research Committee approval and thus stopped a student many years of study in a way that so far is similar to what we associate with corruption and mafia methods. This happened with an instruction outside the formally correct organs. Buen explained to me on the phone that NKKs Director, Marianna Ono Njøten was not familiar with the case, and that she could confirm that it neither had been discussed in a board meeting.

Buen was referred to the editor, who said she had received instructions directly, given her past both the Board and the CEO. She had been instructed not to tell who gave her instructions.

Parallel to these events the "political highest level" had begun their campaign for the parliamentary elections in September 2013. Prime Minister Jens Stoltenberg began his campaign by telling the Norwegian people on the news that under the coalition government survival of cancer had increased from 1 out of 2 to 2 out of 3[104]. That the Prime Minister and the Minister of Health on many occasions, inadvertently I believe, has provided the population with data that contradict facts about the Norwegian cancer care, is serious. The question is therefore whether the population, now that the Cancer Registry's 50-year practice of discretion paint is discovered, will get to know the truth? My impression of Stoltenberg as person is that whatever position after the election he will have, he will correct the mistake and also take seriously what this means for cancer diseased Norwegians.

August 2013
July passed while Buen butted in a wall of silence. The excitement about who was behind the obstruction of the dog experiment fell in

line with the realisation that we might never know *who* and *why*, or *what* or *who* was behind this person again.

Irritated by this secrecy in violation of the Administration laws, but not sure how I should relate to the Prime Minister's election campaign initiative, I contacted one of Vestfold's most experienced county politicians, Ivar Ramberg, which I hoped knew me well enough that the amazing story I had to tell, had a chance to be believed.

Ramberg believed me. What was more, he answered my long story with such a good proposal that radically changed my original plan. Instead of the ambition to reach decision makers in Parliament and the Ministry of Health through the publication, Ramberg's proposal had as a consequence that the publication could be an element in an already initiated political process. That the purpose of the book publication can be achieved even before it is available to the public. He envisioned a first concentrated information conveyed to a non-party political group consisting of health politically motivated members of parliament from both blue-blue and red-green side.

Ramberg predicted that the likely new government after the election would at least need the first one hundred days to warm up the new seats and come so close to the resting heart rate that those who in his opinion ought to get the first information was sufficiently motivated to spend time on it.

Little over a week after meeting with Ramberg Thoresen sent me the following e-mail with the title "Hmmm":

> "One of my cancer patients who went to the Hospital in Vestfold, and that came to me after the hospital had given her up, got this answer to her question whether she could try acupuncture, "Yes, that's fine, but do not go to Thoresen, for he has already killed several people.""

After having unravelled this it showed that the source of this "information" is one I know and recognise as an absolutely reliable person. Both she, her friend, the patient and the physician who made

266

this statement about his "competitor", must be in the interest of the patient remain anonymous.

September 2013
Buen has not yet given up to know more about *who* and *why*, and will await to proceed with the case because she feels insecure as to whether "someone" will also put pressure on FDU to overturn the approval of the experiment. Insecurity was no less after the last e-mail she received from the manager of the NKK´s Board.

> "NKK has received many responses that we front such an attempt at a potentially life-threatening disorder that mammary tumours are. We therefore found after a detailed assessment not to disclose information about your project.
>
> Sincerely
> Siv Sandø"

The explanation from Chairman Sandø is strange. Considering that NKK declined to disseminate information about the dog experiment, *no other than those directly involved should have knowledge of this*. Yet she writes "NKK has received *many reactions* [my italics] [...]". Therefore, I ask myself: Who did these "many reactions" come from - if they exist (?) - and where have these people the information about the dog experiment from?

In the absence of an acceptable dialogue with NKK Buen sends a request to the Veterinary Association regarding a description of the experiment in the Veterinary Journal. Also here Buen is meeting a closed door. How I've got this referenced, the chairman of the Veterinary Association professional advice, Ellef Blakstad, raised the "ethical banner" (see Chapter 15: "Ethics and Economics in cancer treatment") and argued against Buen that it would be ethically questionable to advertise such an attempt[105].

We have reached 15th of September. Just before the experiment should have been initiated, I ask Thoresen describe other similar experiences he wants included in the book:

> • Preparations for a dog trial at the Veterinary College was planned on the basis of a scholarship I had received from the Cancer Society, was stopped without explanation.
> • A planned doctoral program at the University of Nottingham, who conducted tests on the peptides that are found in the blood of a breast cancer patient, was cancelled. At the same time I get a message that their laboratory technician accidentally come to destroy our remaining inventory of the peptides.
> • Via Thomas Grammel, one of my contacts in Germany, where I teach the method several times a year, I came in contact with the University Hospital of Halle. They have a department for breast cancer for women, where thorough feasibility studies have shown not to have any effect of chemotherapy. The professional management wanted to try my method on these patients, and a plan was made for a trial over one year. Just before we were to start, I received an email from the hospital that the experiment was stopped. Grammel has a sister who works in that department. She conveyed that the professors were told from the "highest level" to stop the experiment, without justification.

30th of September

Thoresen calls and says that FDU has come forward again, but now with the "opposite" attitude. It was about that "someone" in FDU had demanded changes in the ad Buen had commissioned in Dog Sports as compensation for the loss of editorial coverage in the magazine and on NKKs Facebook page. Via editor Horakova Buen got presented a paraphrase of the advertisement that transformed it from giving a positive image of the attempt to have a deterrent effect on dog owners. At the same time a recommendation was introduced into the ad to *use a method other than the what ad originally was going to disclose, namely operation.* Recommendation consisted of a claim that surgery has a good prognosis, *which it in no way has. It is precisely because of the poor prognosis of this method* and the urgent need for effective curative cancer treatment that Buen wanted to conduct the experiment.

From their website I read that FDU is a state agency with limited work and responsibility: "NARA will ensure that the necessary use of laboratory animals is conducted in accordance with animal welfare regulations".

This description indicates that the boundaries of FDUs competence and jurisdiction are drawn far beyond what I can see has something to do with safeguarding animal welfare in the experimental context. In practice, such an intervention will be tantamount to a complete withdrawal of the approval. That it is done in such a way I believe is because that there is no good reason to overturn the approval to rejection of the application. Together with the reconsideration from NKK and the Veterinary Association's response the obstacles may have by now have become so high and broad that they are not to be either jumped or gotten around.

Unlike NKK and the Veterinary Association FDU has at least provided a justification for its intervention in the dog experiment. However, the impression I have formed of a brutal override of norms, laws and regulations only furthered by the FDU believe them entitled to edit the ad because Buen has included in the ad text that FDU has approved the experiment.

15th of November
In a full-page ad in Morgenbladet Moan figures as *superstar Johan Moan* - with fashionable sunglasses. The ad is placed by the NAR in a campaign with the motto "With brainpower the future will be created"[106].

6th of February 2014

I just heard a recording of Dagsnytt Eighteen of 31st of January 2014, where this years GP in 2010, Jørgen Skavland, outbids Stoltenberg with regard to the progress in the Norwegian cancer care[107].

From Thoresen I received this morning an sms regarding the article "Targovax-emission" in the Finance newspaper, which tells of "Prime results with cancer vaccine" and "Peptidebased immunotherapy that teaches the immune system itself to fight cancer", which Thoresen has done for 30 years.

I have for some time also known about a trip he made between lectures at Murdoch University in Australia in December 2013 and hospitals in Haifa after the New Year, a trip to a country I do not get to name before the next book. The conclusion I can write is that in this country dedicated people have began recruiting dogs to assist in the completion of Buen´s dog trials at Telemark University College.

Appendix

19. Sergio Manzetti´s epitome of the laboratory research

20. Excerpt from an article about Are Thoresen´s treatment method

21. Thoresen´s clinical study

22. Michael Greenwood: "Cancer and the Hidden Tradition – Is There a Role for Acupuncture Beyond Adjunctive"

270

19. Sergio Manzetti´s epitome of the laboratory research

The first attempt is cantered around the unusually high content of a variety of blood fractions that were centrifuged in October 2003. These fractions were extracted from a volunteer who was treated with LV3 by Thoresen. The sample showed significant changes in the content. These changes have not been compared to an untreated person, but the assumption that the changes are too large for a standard serological situation under non-affected circumstances, these graphs were the start of further investigation of acupuncture stimulus' effect on blood content.

The blood tests of a cancer patient that was donated and taken before and after treatment (60 seconds) was the object of study. Via reverse-phase HPLC there were no changes found in the sample before and after acupuncture, but using a strong cationic HPLC a fraction was found that prior to acupuncture were normal, and after the stimulus increased in signal by about 20X in HPLC-plot area. This fraction was assayed for protein content. The results showed an increase of 0.54 mg/l before and after acupuncture. This was submitted for MS/MS "peptide fingerprinting" in order to examine whether the content was feasible for sequencing. The contents were sequenced to 72 possible peptide candidates, ranked statistically. 12 of these candidates were chosen from statistical probability since they were part of cancer-related proteins.

The synthesis of these 12 peptides gave an opportunity to test these peptides in different cells.

Of the cells tested, the peptides gave the most impact on breast cancer cell MCF7. The results from one of the leading cancer research laboratories in the United States, Charles River Laboratories, Ann Arbor, Michigan, showed an effect by these peptides on both cellular cell growth and partly to slow tumour growth of the MCF7-type in mice without immune systems.

An RNA-chip test, where expressed RNA from MCF7-cells was identified before and after application of the 12 peptides showed actual results of cell growth inhibitory character[108].

More details from the laboratory tests are included in the article below. (My note).

20. Excerpt from an article about Are Thoresen´s treatment method

"Changes in the blood after the described treatment. Identification and isolation of pharmacopotential bioactive peptides from the human body, and their preliminary application against breast cancer"

I have shown and detected 12 bioactive peptides with strong anti-cancer activity. The peptides were isolated from the blood of a human patient with breast cancer treated by acupuncture, re-synthesized and tested against several breast cancer cell types, 1 colon cancer cell type, a prostate cancer cell type and a healthy-cell line model. The effect of the peptides resulted to 100 % cell death on the most common breast cancer cell type, MCF7, after 96 hours. The speed of cell-death was shown to be equivalent to other drugs as Tamoxifen and Doxorubicin, however differing from Doxorubicin and Tamoxifen which are highly toxic and extinguished 87 % per cent of the healthy cell line model, the peptides seemed to stimulate slightly the growth of the healthy cell lines and induce not harm them. The peptides were recently tested on the common MCF7 cell line in nude mice models, and showed to induce a linear cell-death signal. The relationship between the cell tests and the mice tests suggests that the peptides have a full cell-death effect on MCF7 cells, which however needs to be protected against the immune system of a multicellular organism. The protective method of PEG-modulation is under testing on mice, and will, as expected from other studies performed with PEG, prolong the half-life of the peptides in circulation, and thereby induce stronger cell-death signal to function as a complete pharmacoactive agent.

Results
Sample results and peptides found in the patient

The acupuncture stimulus of the patient yielded a pair of samples, where samples A, from before acupuncture had half the amount of peptides than sample B, from after acupuncture. This instigated not only the rapid effect of generation of changes in the blood after only 60 seconds of acupuncture stimulus, but also a myriad of potential peptides responsible for the internal response to the acupuncture. The key to the isolation process was a sequential choosing of crucial factors, which were not only statistically probable of being in the sample of the diseased woman, but also to be related to some known factors, such as Tumour Necrosis Growth factor as an example. Out of the 70–110 peptides resulting from two different identification methods, 12 were chosen based on their statistical probability of being present in the blood. The probability ranged from 95 %–90 % for 11 of these, and 72 % for one particular. The common theme of all the peptides found, was that they were fragments of proteins, suggesting a mechanism of generation of potential "medical" peptides, from existing proteins in circulation.

Many of the peptides found turned out to be related to cell-cycle regulation proteins. The proteins involved in cell-cycle up and down-regulate cell-growth, and play key roles in daily maintenance and control of the organisms' adaptation to internal and external changes. Table 1 illustrates the origin of the 12 peptides.

Table 4. *List of parent proteins of the 12 peptides originating from subject treated by acupuncture.*

Protein	Statistical Probability	Function
Chain C, Hemoglobin Thionville Alpha Chain Mutant [*H. Sapiens*]	95 %	Oxygen-carrier

Chain A Deoxy hemoglobin [*H. Sapiens*]	93 %	Oxygen-carrier
Glutamyl Prolyl tRna synthetase [*R. Norvegicus*]	95 %	Aminoacid synthesis
Zinc finger, SWIM domain containing [*H. Sapiens*]	95 %	Forming nucleoprotein complex in apoptosis possibly involved with proteasome-Ub pathway [45].
Golgin 45 (JEM-1) leucine zipper nuclear factor [*H. Sapiens*]	93 %	DNA-binding protein first found in leukaemia cases, role in cell maturation [46]
unnamed protein product [*H. Sapiens*]	77 %	Liver-secreted protease inhibitor, antichymotrypsin-like *******
KIAA0476 protein [*H. Sapiens*]	95 %	Unknown factor, detected first in brain tissue. [48]
Winged helix domain-containing isoform B [*H. Sapiens*]	95 %	Possibly involved in chromatin-interactions [49]

unnamed protein product [*H. Sapiens*]	82 %	mRNA from NT2 neuronal precursor cells treated 2-weeks mitotic inhibitor after 5-weeks retinoic acid (RA) induction (unpublished)
Regulatory Protein [*R. Norvegicus*]	95 %	novel mitogenic regulatory gene which is transcriptionally suppressed in cells [50]
Laminin gamma 1 [*M. Musculus*]	94 %	a novel transmembrane protein with a strong and developmentally regulated expression in the nervous system.[51]
Chain A, Nmr Structure Of The Nalp1 P Apoptosis related [*H. Sapiens*]	93 %	Apoptosis inducer – new member of death domain superfamily since 2003[52]

Cytostatic effects on cancer cells

The 12 peptides were tested at Molecular Imaging Laboratories, Ann Arbor, MI, USA. The peptides effect was focused on the most common breast cancer cell type, MCF7. The MCF7 cell line originates from a patient that had breast cancer with spreading to the lungs and bones and is a common cell type to test both commercial and experimental drugs on. The peptides were synthesised at the Biomedical Genomic Centre at the University of Minnesota, and shipped to MIR for testing. At MIR laboratories, the peptides were mixed in an equal dose into a complete mixture, to simulate the acupuncture stimulus, and prepared for application on the cell-plates. The cell-death effect of the peptides has been observed already within the first 24 hours (as seen from results from earlier tests at the University of Massachusetts) to be even faster than the common drug Tamoxifen. After 96 hours, of daily doses, the breast cancer cells are 100 % extinguished (see Fig 1). The effect of the peptide mixture I denoted to have an IC50 of 70. This number delineates its potency. The effect was observed as a hyperbolic curve, where the highest concentrations give the fastest effect of cancer-cell death.

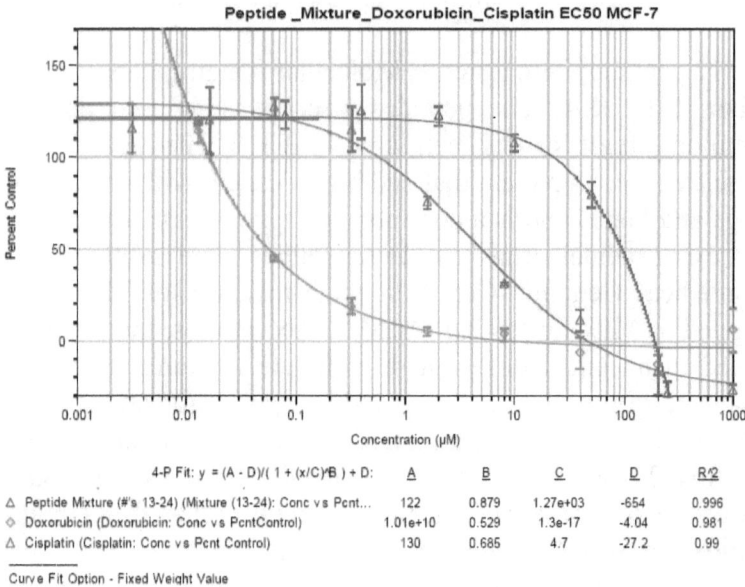

Peptide _Mixture_Doxorubicin_Cisplatin EC50 MCF-7

4-P Fit: y = (A - D)/(1 + (x/C)^B) + D:

	A	B	C	D	R^2
△ Peptide Mixture (#'s 13-24) (Mixture (13-24): Conc vs Pcnt...	122	0.879	1.27e+03	-654	0.996
◇ Doxorubicin (Doxorubicin: Conc vs PcntControl)	1.01e+10	0.529	1.3e-17	-4.04	0.981
△ Cisplatin (Cisplatin: Conc vs Pcnt Control)	130	0.685	4.7	-27.2	0.99

Curve Fit Option - Fixed Weight Value

Fig 4. _Determination of the effect of peptide mixture (Dec 08)._

The effect of the complete peptide mixture on the MCF7 breast cancer cell line. The green line shows the effect of the peptide mixture reaching a 100 % cell death at a daily dose of approximately 250uM. The orange and brown lines shows the effect of Doxorubincin and Cisplatin, two regular medicines, which kill the cells starting from lower concentrations (however inducing severe side effect on the patient).

The effect of the 12 peptides shows also another positive aspect, it spares healthy cell lines, _in vitro._ The peptides were tested at the University of Nottingham on a healthy cell line, and show not to harm its growth (see Fig 2). So simultaneously as the peptide mixture kills 100 % of breast cancer cells MCF7, its saves the healthy cell from its killing effect. The potential drug is therefore appearing as selective, and may be related to its origin from the body, resulting from a stimulus of acupuncture.

280

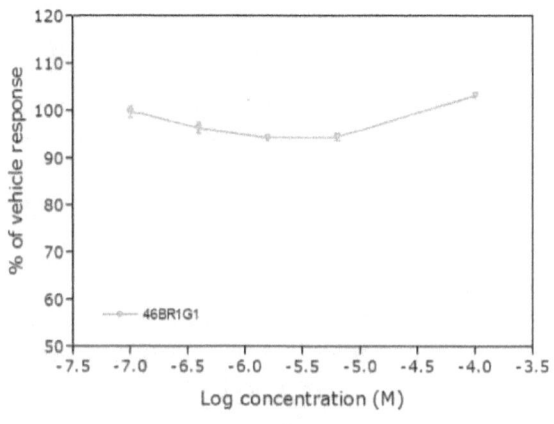

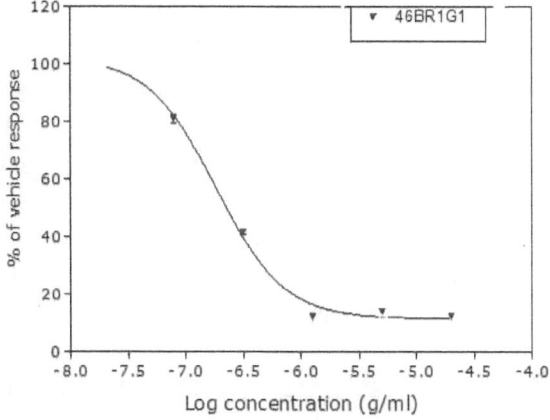

Fig 5. Effects on healthy cell line studies (Aug 08). *Left: The twelve*
peptides did not induce substantial effects on a healthy cell line model
(study from Nottingham University). Right: The regular drug,
Doxorubicin, induced an 87 % death rate on the healthy cell line
model.

The twelve peptides were pilot-tested against an implanted MCF7 tumour in mice at Molecular Imaging Laboratories in September 08. The peptides' chemical structure was in this experiment in unprotected and natural state, which is a regular form to test for efficiency first. Once the results of the peptides in a natural state are interpreted, their effect can be eventually increased by adding a chemical protection.

The mice were injected with three doses of peptides, 20mg/kg, 40mg/kg and 80mg/kg peptide. The injection was given daily for a period of 21 days, and the effect was visible: the highest dose gave the strongest cancer-growth retardation, the middle dose gave a lower cancer growth-retardation and the lowest dose gave the weakest anti-cancer effect (See Fig 3). The results show that the peptides have a preserved effect in mice which follows a dose-dependent scheme. Additionally, the results show that the peptides act strongest through the blood and not when injected directly in the tumour. However, the potency of the effect must be strengthened and the central option is to prolong their endurance in circulation. The method for doing this is through a so called PEG-ligation technology. Our contractor, Cresalus Inc, Kentucky USA, have in early February completed the synthesis of 240 mg of PEG-protected peptides. Molecular Imaging Laboratories are initiating the testing of PEG peptides on mice in the middle of February and results are awaited by the beginning of March 09.

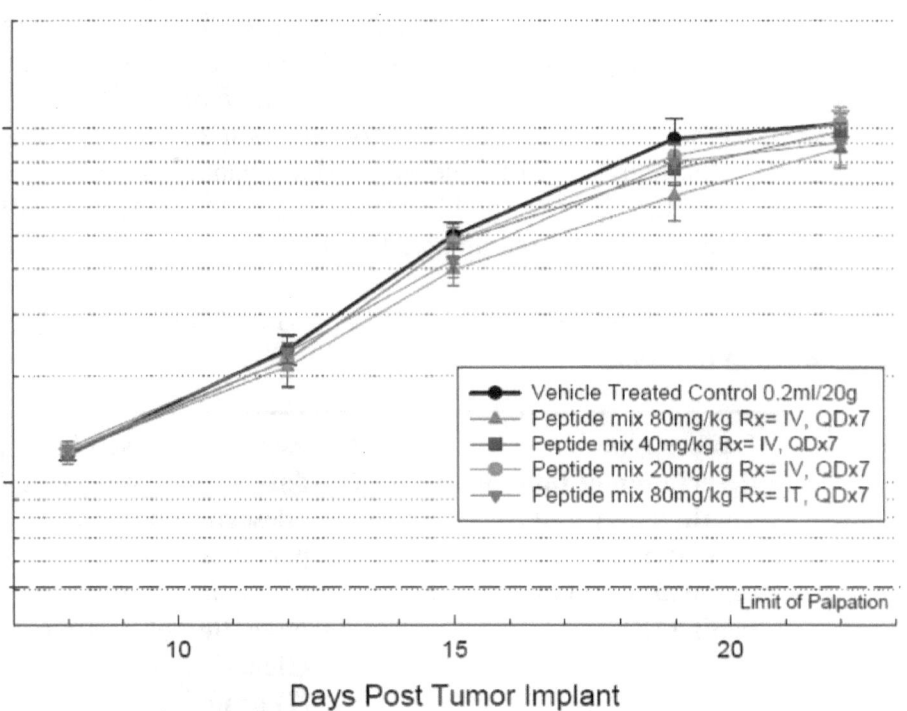

Fig 6. Peptides effect on mice models in unprotected formulation. The five lines show the growth of the tumour in five groups of mice that were treated in alternative ways. The black line illustrates the mice that were carrying an MCF7 tumour and did not receive any medication. The red line shows the mice that carried a tumour and were given 80mg/kg of peptide mixture, showing the slowest tumour growth. The blue line shows the growth of the tumour in the mice receiving half dose, 40mg/kg, showing a stronger tumour growth. The pink line shows the growth of the tumour in the mice receiving the lowest dose of peptides, 20mg/kg. The green line shows the growth of the tumour in mice receiving the highest dose injected in the tumour.

21. Thoresen´s clinical study

Table 1. On the request of Dr. Med. Ottestad, Chief Medical Officer of the mammary cancer department at the Radium Hospital of Norway, I carefully noted and measured all human patients during a certain time span between *April 22nd 2003 and January 26th 2004; they were not "cherry-picked" to show the best outcomes.* These notes are the foundation of table nr. 1. These human patients were diagnosed by their doctor, and I have just accepted the diagnosis. All patients have been followed up until 01.01.2010 (or until they died).

Table 1: Summary of my treatment protocols and their interim outcomes in humans

#	Cancer type / description of tumour / malignancy and indication of malignant (M) or benign (B)	Patient, year of birth)	Acupoint(s) used / date of first treatment / description of progression or development and indication of positive effect (P), uncertain (?) or negative (N)
1.	Aggressive mammary carcinoma / malignant **(M)**	Woman, born 1962	LV03 / 19/11-02 / the cancer was operated and treated with medication, but the hospital gave up and sent her home to die. After treatments every month she lived for 4 years, and then died during a few weeks. **(P)**

2.	Prostate cancer: with multiple skeletal metastases / malignant (**M**)	Man, born 1942	HT09 + TH02 / September –02 / after starting the acupuncture treatment the cancer has gone "dormant". The situation is stable. PSA = 0.35. No other treatment has been performed (**P**)
3.	Leukaemia / benign (**B**)	Man, born 1944	SI18 & LU01 / 18/6-03 / the blood-values have been stable since the treatment started (**P**)
4.	Mammary carcinoma / 6 mm. tumour on left side / malignant (**M**)	Woman, born 1945	LV03 / 18/6-03 / she was not operated or given any other form of treatment by the hospital. The tumour went almost totally away, and can now not be detected (P)
5.	Uterine cervical cancer Stage IIIB: / malignant (**M**)	Woman, born 1958	TH02 / 30/7-03 / diagnosed in spring 2002. After treatment with acupuncture the cancer has disappeared completely (**P**)

6.	Renal carcinoma / started in the right kidney with metastases in the liver where 6 metastases can be seen / malignant (**M**)	Man, born 1922	HT09 / 17/9-03 / after two treatments the man did not come, and I later learned that he had died. (**N**)
7.	Melanosarcoma / lateral side of the arm, / malignant (**M**)	Woman, born 1932	HT09 (as the cancer was situated on the LI-meridian) / 1/10-03 / the patient seem to get better and better, and then suddenly died 14. January 2004. (**N**)
8.	Mammary carcinoma / 20 mm. tumour in left breast. Operated 10/2-99. Then metastases to liver and the skeleton. Also now multiple cancers in the right breast / malignant (**M**)	Woman, born 1957	LV03 / 28/10-03 / she was not operated or given any other form of treatment by the hospital after the discovery of the metastases and the recurrence of the breast cancer. All tumours started to shrink, then halted, and are now static. (**P**)

9.	Mammary carcinoma / 18 mm. tumour on left side / malignant (**M**)	Woman, born 1964	LV03 / 24/11-03 / she was operated and given additional treatment to stop metastases. Treatment to prevent metastases. (**?**)
10.	Dysplasia of the glossal epithelium / cell-changes on the tongue / benign (**B**)	Woman, born 1950	KI03 / 7/10-03 / the patient has received no other treatment, and the cell-changes are stable (**P**)
11.	Colon carcinoma / operated / malignant (**M**)	Man, born 1930	HT09 / 22/10-03 / treatment to prevent the cancer from metastasing or reappearing (**?**)
12.	Mammary carcinoma of the left breast / the carcinoma was ca. 1, cm in diameter / malignant (**M**)	Woman, born 1950	LV03 / 8/12-03 / the woman had undergone surgery and the cancer + 14 lymph-nodes were excised. The treatment was performed for prevention. No other treatment after the surgery is performed (**?**)
13.	Chronic myelo-monocytic leukaemia / benign (**B**)	Woman, born 1947	LV03 / 19/11-03 / no obvious change in the blood-values after start of acupuncture treatment (**?**)

14.	Chronic diarrhoea after former radiation of cancer / this is not a cancer treatment, but only damage after radiation	Woman, born 1948	PC05 + KI0+3 / 19/11-03 / the diarrhoea disappeared after 4 weeks and 2 treatments. Has stayed Ok since then **(P)**
15.	Brain cancer / inoperable / half of it benign, half malignant **(B + M)**	Woman, born 1964	TH05 + PC08 / 22/12-03 / since treatment started the patient has been stable **(P)**
16.	Mammary carcinoma, aggressive type, right side with multiple metastases / malignant **(M)**	Woman, born 1960	LV03 / 18/6-03 / she was not operated or given any other form of treatment by the hospital, as the doctors considered the case incurable. Since the treatment started, there has been no growth of the cancer or the metastases **(P)**
17.	Carcinoma of the prostate / malignant **(M)**	Man, born 1954	BL40 / 15/1-04 / operated additionally with cryo-technique, difficult to evaluate **(?)**

| 18 | Mammary carcinoma, aggressive. Operated, but after operation metastases to the liver and the skeleton malignant (**M**) | Woman, born 1945 | LV03 / 26/1-03 / after the treatment started there was a stop in the growth of the cancer (**P**) |

Table 2. On the request of Dr. Med. Ottestad, Chief Medical Officer of the mammary cancer department at the Radium Hospital of Norway, I carefully noted and measured all veterinary patients during a certain time span between *April 22nd 2003 and January 26th 2004; they were not "cherry-picked" to show the best outcomes.* These notes are the foundation of table nr. 2. These veterinary patients were mostly diagnosed by myself, with fine needle biopsy, but some came with the diagnosis from other veterinarians. All patients have been followed up until 31.12.2009 (or until they died).

Table 2: Summary of my treatment protocols and their interim outcomes in animals

#	Cancer type / description of tumour / malignancy and indication of malignant (M) or benign (B)	Patient, year of birth	Acupoint (s) used / date of first treatment / description ofprogression or development and indication of positive effect (P), uncertain (?) or negative (N)
1	Mammary carcinoma / 10 & 8 mm tumours in both sides / malignant (M)	Female dog, Chihuahua, born 1999	LV03 / 22/4-03 / the tumours went almost totally away, then reappeared, and are now stabile. No other treatment (P)

2	Perianal tumour / 12 cm. Diameter / benign (**B**)	Female dog, Chihuahua, born 1999	CV23 / spring –02 / the tumour was stable for 1 year, started then to grow autumn –03, and the dog was put down in November –03. No other treatment (**N**)
3	Osteosarcoma left front leg / 11 cm^2 / malignant (**M**)	Dog, mixed breed, born 1994	HT09 / November –02 / in April –03 the cancer was totally gone. No other treatment (**P**)
4	Carcinoma of the endothelium of the abdomen, with metastases to several organs / malignant (**M**)	Male dog, Riesenschnauser, born 1989	SP06 / 1. April –03 / the first 3 months everything seem to go better, but then the dog suddenly died in august. No other treatment (**N**)
5	Mammary tumour: diameter 1.1 cm / benign (**B**)	Bitch, English setter, born 1996	LV03 / 17/7-03 / After one year the tumor was totally gone. No other treatment has been performed (**P**)

6	Mammary tumours (2): diameter 1.4 cm, 1,1 cm / benign (B)	Bitch, English setter, born 1998	LV03 / 17/7-03 / After one year the tumors are 0,3 and 0,2 mm. No other treatment has been performed (P)
7	Carcinoma of the epithelium / 4 cm. right front paw / malignant (M)	Male dog, Riesenschnauser, born 1994	KI01 / 15/7-03 / the carcinoma was operated before I saw the dog, but had spread to right back leg and right axilla / after treatment the cancer was reduced with 60 %. No other treatment has been performed (P)
8	Seminoma / Left testis 7.5 cm diameter / benign (B)	Male dog, Golden retriever, born 1988	LU11 / 17/6-03 / the tumour stopped growing, and has stayed stable since. No other treatment has been performed (P)

9	Chondrosarcoma / left side of abdomen, 12 x 12 cm / malignant (**M**)	Male dog, Mixed breed, born 1995	LU11 & LU01 / 22/7-03 / after each treatment the cancer shrunk with 20 % during 1 week, but then started to grow again. This pattern has repeated itself after every treatment. Now the cancer is 17 x 20 cm. (**? P**)
10	Lymphosarcoma / have been treated for a long time with cortisone / malignant (**M**)	Male dog, Norwegian hare-hound, born 1996	LV03 / 10/9-03 / 2 days after the first treatment the dog was acutely worse, and was put down by the owner (**N**)
11	Mammary carcinoma / multiple tumours in both sides, size varYing between 5 mm to 20 mm. / malignant (**M**)	Icelandic sheep-dog bitch, born 2001	LV03 / 30/9-03 / she was not operated or given any other form of treatment. The tumours went almost totally away, and can now not be detected (**P**)

12	Malignant mesenchymal tumour at the inside of the knee / 10 cm. diameter / malignant (**M**)	Male dog, mixed breed, born 1999	LU11 / 10/10-03 / after the first treatment the cancer has stopped to grow and seem to be stable. (**P**)
13	Epithelial carcinoma over the ischium / 5 x 4 cm / malignant (**M**)	Bitch, big poodle, born 1992	SP01 + HT09 / 28/10-03 / after treatment started the cancer has shrunk to 1.9 x 1.9 cm. No other medication or treatments have been performed (**P**)
14	Mastocytoma / malignant (**M**)	Male dog, English setter, born 1997	HT09 / 20/12-03 / after start of treatment the cancer is reduced by approximately 70 % (**P**)

| 15 | Mammary carcinoma on left side; operated but had metastases; new cancer is developing on the right side / malignant (**M**) | Bitch, Tibetan temple dog, born 1991 | LV03 bilateral / 20/1-03 / since the treatment started the tumour is somewhat reduced (**P**)#2 |

Results

Table 3: Summary of my treatment protocols and their interim outcomes in 34 patients (all patients during one year)

Clinical outcome [interim]	*Number of Cases*
Humans	18
Dogs	15
Horses	1
Total Benign tumors	8
Total Malign tumors	26
Reduced growth in benign tumors	2
Reduced growth in malign tumors	12

Total disappearance of visible benign tumors	2
Total disappearance of visible malign tumors	4
Overall positive development in number of benign tumors	4
Overall negative development in number of benign tumors	1
Overall positive development in number of malign cancer	18
Overall negative development in number of malign cancer	5
Number of patient impossible to say is positive or negative due to massive treatment in the hospital, or total removal of the cancer surgically.	6
Number of patients that died during the treatment	5

References:
- Chumakov AM, Miller CW, Chen DL, Koeffler HP. Analysis of p53 transactivation through high-affinity binding sites. Oncogene. 1993 Nov;8(11):3005–11.
- Cinar B, Koeneman KS, Edlund M, Prins GS, Zhau HE, Chung LW. Androgen receptor mediates the reduced tumor growth, enhanced androgen responsiveness, and selected

target gene transactivation in a human prostate cancer cell line. Cancer Res. 2001 Oct 1;61(19):7310–7.

- Deppert W. The Yin and Yang of p53 in cellular proliferation.Semin Cancer Biol. 1994 Jun;5(3):187–202. Review.

- Ekeland T.-J., Placebofenomenet – hvordan kan det forstås, Tidsskr. Nor. Lægeforen. 2000;120:3017–20.

- Johnson JM, Harrod R, Franchini G.(2001). Molecular biology and pathogenesis of the human T-cell leukaemia/lymphotropic virus Type-1 (HTLV-1). Int J Exp Pathol. 82: 135–47.

- Kim KJ, Lee MW, Choi JH, Sung KJ, Moon KC, Koh JK. (2002). Abstract CD30-positive T-cell-rich pseudolymphoma induced by gold acupuncture. Br J Dermatol. 146: 882–4.

- Kurono Y, Egawa M, Yano T, Shimoo K. (2002). The effect of acupuncture on the coronary arteries as evaluated by coronary angiography: a preliminary report. Am J Chin Med.30: 387–96.

- Lewis DL, Hagstrom JE, Loomis AG, Wolff JA, Herweijer H. Efficient delivery of siRNA for inhibition of gene expression in postnatal mice. Nat Genet. 2002 Sep;32(1):107–8. Epub 2002 Jul 29.

- Loeppky RN, Goelzer P. Microsome-mediated oxidation of N-nitrosodiethanolamine (NDELA), a bident carcinogen. Chem Res Toxicol. 2002 Apr;15(4):457–69.

- Lu H. C., A complete translation of the Yellow Emperors classic of internal medicine and the difficult classic, translated from the Chinese, The academy of oriental Heritage, Vancouver, Canada, 1978.

- Maoshing N. (1995). The Yellow Emperor's Classic of Medicine. A New translation of the Neijing Suwen with commentary. Shambhala Publications Inc, Boston.

- Miller C, Koeffler HP.(1993).P53 mutations in human cancer. Leukemia. 1993 Suppl 2: 18–21.

- Miller DK. The role of the Caspase family of cysteine proteases in apoptosis.Semin Immunol. 1997 Feb;9(1):35–49. Review.
- Pohorille A. et al., Membrane peptides and their role in protobiological evolution. Orig Life Evol Biosph. 2003 Apr;33(2):173–97.
- Rogers PA, Schoen AM, Limehouse J. (1992). Acupuncture for immune-mediated disorders. Literature review and clinical applications. Probl. Vet. Med. 4:162–93.
- Shen J, Glaspy J. (2001). Acupuncture: evidence and implications for cancer supportive care. Cancer Pract. 9:147–50.
- Tagliaferri M, Cohen I, Tripathy D. (2001). Complementary and alternative medicine in early-stage breast cancer. Semin. Oncol. 28:121–34.
- Sherr CJ. (2000–2001). Cell cycle control and cancer. Harvey Lect. 96:73–92.
- Thoresen A., Akupunkturbehandling av Equint Sarcoid, Norsk Veterinærtidsskrift, 1995 *107,* 10.
- Thoresen A, Veterinærmedisin, Komplementære og Alternative metoder, pp.442–445, ISBN 82–994172–4–4, 621 pages. English edition; ISBN 82–994172–2–8, gages 358–363.
- Udagawa N. The mechanism of osteoclast differentiation from macrophages: possible roles of T lymphocytes in osteoclastogenesis. J Bone Miner Metab. 2003;21(6):337–43.
- Yang Q, Wesch H, Mueller KM, Bartsch H, Wegener K, Hollstein M. (2000). Analysis of radon-associated squamous cell carcinomas of the lung for a p53 gene hotspot mutation. Br J Cancer. 82: 763–6.

22. Michael Greenwood: "Cancer and the Hidden Tradition – Is There a Role for Acupuncture Beyond Adjunctive"

http://www.paradoxpublishing.com/assets/files/publications/articles/aama/vol-23-1-cancer.pdf

In the second half of the article, from page 45, there are descriptions with reference to Thoresen´s treatment method.

To reprint the article one must obtain the author and the journal's consent. I have chosen to let the ones with special interests retrieve the article on you're their own pc through the link. They may also print it for non-commercial use.
(My note).

23. Some examples of the method's distribution

The first three examples are feedback from the time around the final editing of the manuscript, around the turn of 2013/14. Followed by diverse responses to an inquiry Thoresen in 2010 at my request he sent some of his foreign colleagues who utilizes his treatment method.

The first e-mail was forwarded to me in connection with Thoresen is a guest lecturer at Murdoch University in Fremantle, Australia, at the invitation of Professor Bruce Ferguson. It was originally sent to Ferguson by one of his own pupils, ie a second-generation student of Are Thoresen.

Sent from my iPad
Bruce Ferguson, DVM, MS
President, American Association of TCVM
Vice-President, World Association of TCVM
www.naturalvet.org
www.tcvm.com.au

Begin forwarded message:
From:
Date: 6 December 2013 8:18:22 am AWST
To: naturalvet@earthlink.net
Subject: Sarcoid success!

Hi Bruce,
I hope you are well and that 2013 has been a great year for you. I would just like to share a success story that I have had with sarcoids in a horse.
Denny is a 7 year old quarterhorse mare with a 4 year history of multiple sarcoids. We have tried a number of different treatments with Denny over the years, including surgery, xxterra and fluoride paste, all with limited success.
I thought I would apply Dr Are Thorenson's 1 needle technique to this case and the results have been amazing.
3 of Denny's sarcoids are located on the Stomach Channel. I treated her 2 weeks ago with 1 dry-needle at LIV 1 for 20min.

300

These attached results are from two weeks post treatment. The sarcoids are now 30 % of their original size. The owner is really happy!

Thanks to you, Marisa and your fantastic course Bruce!

Kind Regards,
Dr. E. B. BSc BVMS
Coral Coast Veterinary Hospital
12 Bassett Way Carnarvon WA 6701

Ph: (08) 99411155
Fax: (08) 99411166

This email's authenticity can be verified directly by the stated personalia.

oOo

From: J. K.-A. .]
Sent: 24. desember 2013 20:05
To: Are Thoresen
Subject: Re: The lady from Costa Rica

Dear Dr. Thoresen,
Your treatment worked! I have had no treatment by the western-medical people, just your treatment on June 3rd and some tuning-up acupuncture by L. Z. I had a rectoscopy last week, Dec. 16, and the T1 is so tiny the doctor almost didn't find it and hasn't even sized it, but said in his report, paraphrasing from the Spanish: the exophytic lesion is many dimensions less than previously observed; towards the top margin in tretrovision a decrease in the extent of the lesion was observed. The biopsy says: anal intraepithelial high grade lesion/carcinoma in situ.
It's shrinking, just like you said it would.
Thankyouthankyouthankyouthankyou.
I can't tell you how happy my husband and I are – you are a true and unique asset to health.
Should I have a follow-up treatment with you?
The very best to you and yours this holiday season.
Best regards,
J. K.-A.

oOo

Kopi: T. B..
Emne: T. B., Thun, Switzerland

Dear Are Thoresen
First of all we wish you a happy new year 2014!
Please find as an attachment my medical abstract (word document) as well as the E-Mail of my wife including several documents. Please do not hesitate to contact us in case you need more information.

Best regards
R. B.

Gesendet: Samstag, 04. Januar 2014 um 14:39 Uhr
Von: ..
Betreff: Akupunktur

Lieber Are
Hier die Operationsberichte, die 4 oberen Blätter sind von der Operation vom 9. Juli. Nach dieser Operation musste ich 9 Sessionen Chemotherapie machen.
Am 2. und am 4. Oktober war ich bei dir zur Akupunktur.
Am 22. Oktober war die 2. Operation (untere 3 Blätter). Vor der Operation sagten mir die Ärzte, dass sie fast sicher das Stoma noch lassen werden, da sie das vom Krebs befallene Stück Dickdarm herausschneiden müssen. Bei der Operation waren alle sehr erstaunt, dass gar kein Krebs mehr vorhanden war. Sie entfernten mir Uterus, Ovarien, Lymphknoten, Omentum majus und Appendix. Sie konnten das Stoma rückverlegen.
Ich musste noch einmal 9 Sessionen Chemotherapie machen. Ich bin froh, dass mein Bauch nachher richtig heilen kann.
Peter Grob steckt mir jeden Monat die Nadel. Ich bin überzeugt, dass ich dadurch endgültig von diesem Krebs geheilt bin! Vielen herzlichen Dank!!!

Viele liebe Grüsse
T.

This e-mail is followed by six attachments from the treating hospital, confirming the text of the message. The annexes have not been placed in the book, but is found in my archive of underlying documentation.
(My comment)

oOo

Dear Are
I have used your method on 2 patients (lung cancer, vaginal cancer) both old women, seems the results are quite good. I'll be more than happy to help you with your request.

R. R. DM.

oOo

Hi Are:
As I told you I′ve been treating patients with cancer using your method since 2 years ago. I′ve some photos and if you want I can make a summary of these cases.

F. M. DVM.

oOo

Dear Are,
I first heard your cancer treatment in the eariler 90's in Alanta. As my pulse diagnosis has improved my results with your method have gotten better. Significant improvement in most cases, around 80 %. At least it seems to hold the disease at bay for long periods of time. My poorest result is lymphosarcoma. I have used it in probably over 100 cases of cancer during the last decade.

Cheers,
C.L. DVM

oOo

Dear Are.

I am J. M. G. from Barcelona IVAS Course.

I have used your method in one horse with a big lump (biggest than a hen egg) in the sheath with only one neddle in CV meridiam, but not exactly in one acupunture point. I found one depression between CV2 and Bai Hui and I neddle in. In the first session, the lump was reduced at the half. I did five sessions, and the lump was gone completly, I couldn't feel nothing under the skin. It was in July.

At the moment the horse and his sheath are perfect. I send you pictures about.

I hope it can help you.

The best for you
J. M. G.

oOo

Are!

I have treated 12 cases following your method: 6 mammary cancer (bitches): all of them have improved, 3 totally, 3 have received surgical treatment after 4 sessions (when size and inflammtion had reduced) and until now metàstasis or recidives have not been found.

1 intestinal cancer (cat) : no positive results.

1 linfoma (tracheal zone, dog male, Shi-Tzu): its size has been reduced 50 % and dog is healthy after 10 months from begining.

1 peri-anal (Doberman, male): size has reduced 30 % and there's no pain nor bleeding.

1 urinary bladder (Setter, female): good answer during 6 months (no bleeding, no haematuria) and after owner decided euthanasia.

1 scapular osteosarcoma : no answer.

Best regards,
F.

oOo

Dear Are,

in the following I describe a treatment of dog with canine hemangioperizytom.

Dog, Sheparddog-Rottweiler-Mix, 9 years, male, 57 kg 2005-03-30: 1 st investigation of a tumor on the right front leg on the laterodorsal side just proximal to the carpaljoint. The neo was very rigid and had two parts. The main tumor was as large as a half chicken egg, the second a bit more dorsally and just distal to the larger one was like a great bean.

We took a fine-needle-aspiration biopsy and the histoligal result was a localy maligne canine hemangioperizytoma.

We decided that the tumor is related to the HT and/or TH-meridian. We answered by stimulating the controll by needeling KI03 and KI01 once a week.

Ajax accepted sauerkraut and yogurth (great!) and Immundog (Orthovet).

2005-06-05: The tumor did not raise anymore up to now and we made a photo with outline tumorborders.

2005-06-24: The tumor is viewable smaller (the little one not touchable, the larger one just the half of the original size).

2005-08-02: The tumor is gone. We decided to give two sessions in KI-Meridian and then to make a controll FNA – but we could not – because the tumor was gone and we no idea where to place the neddle.

There was no rezidiv until now.

oOo

Lieber Are,

letzten Dienstag war die Kundin wieder in der Klinik Hofheim zum Ultraschall: Kein Tumor mehr zu finden! Die Klinik glaubt nun, sie hätten sich bei Ihrer ersten Diagnose vertan, obwohl angeblich bereits deutlich Wandauflösungen zu sehen waren. Ich habe die Kundin gebeten, mir diese ersten + die Kontroll (nach ca. 6 Wochen) Ultraschallbilder auf CD zu brennen, oder wenigsten als Foto zu besorgen. Sobald ich diese habe, schicke ich dir alles zu!

Fairerweise muss ich Dir sagen, dass ich zunächst mit Deiner Akupunkturmethode gearbeitet habe, und ca. 2 Wochen vor dem Kontrollultraschall nur noch mit Bioresonanz, da ich sie per Akupunktur nicht übertherapieren wollte.

Liebe Grüße
S.

oOo

Summaries of my cancer patients treated with your method:

1.   Weiblicher Mittelschnautzer, "Gipsy" silber, 14 Jahre alt.
Erster Besuch in der Praxis wegen seit 4 Wochen rezidvierender blutiger
Cystitis.
Leukozytose, Blut und Leukos im Urin. Strangurie, Mitrialinsuffizienz,
Arrythmien. Hatte vor kurzem eine Umfangsvermehrung auf dem
Blasenmeridian der entfernt wurde. Hypothyreose : Euthyroxgabe.
Haustierarzt gab Antibiotika und Homöopathika.
Behandlung mit Akupunktur bis 6.4.04 dann Überweisung zum Ultraschall
zur Tierklinik in Hofheim:
Tumor am Blasenhals, Harnröhre wahrscheinlich mitbetroffen. Verdacht
auf Übergangsepithelkarzinom der Blase Rat der Tierklinik: Meatcam, ev
Interleukininfiltration derHarnröhre. Prognose infaust.
    Besitzer gibt 3 Tg Metacam, wurde dann wegen heftigster Druchfälle
    wieder abgesetzt.

Am 16.4.04 mit Tumortherapie/Akupunktur begonnen: ausschließlich
Herz 9, Herzpuls sehr schwach.
In der folgenden Zeit alle 2–3 Wochen Einnadeltheapie: Herz 9. Keine
weiteren Therapieverfahren.

Ultraschallkontrollen durch die Tierklinik Hofheim: 21.5.05: noch 8 mm
verändertes Gewebe und Zubildung am Blasenhals. Weiterhin Verdacht
auf tumoröses Geschenen. Allgemeinbefinden gut.
5.7.04: Zubildung im Bereich des Blasenhalses nicht mehr zu finden.
Verkalkungen der Harnröhre.
4.10.05: Zubildung wieder sichtbar, gegenüber Errstbefund
geringgradig vergrößert.

Gipsy wurde wegen zunehmender Strangurie und Tenesmus dann Mitte
Oktober eingeschläfert.

2.   Weibliche Schäferhündin, "Susi", geb.: 95.
In Behandlung wegen Chronisch degenerativer Myelopathie.
Herzuntersuchung: geringradige Arrhytmien. Zur Abklärung der
Narkosefähigkeit Ultraschalluntersuchung des Herzens in der Tierklinik
Hofheim.

Verdacht auf großes Chemodektom, Stauungserscheiningen im linken Vorhof und Lungenvenen.

Prognose infaust.

Seither, abgesehen von Geriatrika, keine weitere Behandlung außer Einnadelakupunktur alle 3–4 Wochen: je nach Puls meißt Ni 1.

Ultraschallkontrollen alle 8 Wochen: Der Tumor verändert sich nur geringfügig. "Susi´s" chron degenerative Myelopathie verschlechtert sich unter der Behandlung nicht weiter und das Chemodektom beginnt erst zu schrumpfen, dann aber sehr langsam weiterzuwachsen. (Behandlungsbeginn Juli 04 5.5x5.1 cm, blieb bis Juli 05 unter 6x6 cm). Im Juli 05 mußte die Akupunkturbehandlung wegen starker akuter Beschwerden des rechten Knie und Hüftgelenks, der Lebensqualität wegen, umgestellt werden. Daraufhin wurde eine deutliche Umfangsvermehrung auf 8x8 cm festgestellt. Seit September behandele ich wieder nach Pulsdiagnostik und Einnadeltherapie. Eine neue Kontrolle steht aus.

Im Dezember 05 erfreut sich der Hund guter Gesundheit spielt und ist gerne unterwegs. Laut Aussage des Ultraschalldiagnostikers sei es außergewöhnlich, daß ein Chemodektom so langsam wächst.

oOo

Here are some of my my results (in which all has been "cured"):

1. C. K. 62 year old with stage 3 breast cancer. Treated regularly since 1998. Chemo only.
2. B. O.: 50 year old with stage 3 breast cancer.   Treated regularly since 2003. Chemo only.
3. L. Ya.: 72 year old with stage 3 breast cancer. Treated regularly since 1990. No chemo or radiation.
4. B. E.: 54 year old with positive biopsy. Biopsy was negative after 2 treatments. No chemo or radiation.
5. E. J.: 60 year old with stage 3 breast cancer. Treated with chemo only. Treated regularly since 1995.
6. S. K.t: 65 year old with stage one breast cancer. No chemo or readiation. Treated since 2000.

These are the ones off the top of my head.
P.

24. The dog Mighty

The latest feedback from the patient before the script moves on to a final technical correction from the owner of the dog Mighty, which included a photo taken at Are Thoresen´s first treatment.

From: SU . Sent: 29. januar 2014 01:35
To: .
Subject: bilde Mighty og Are

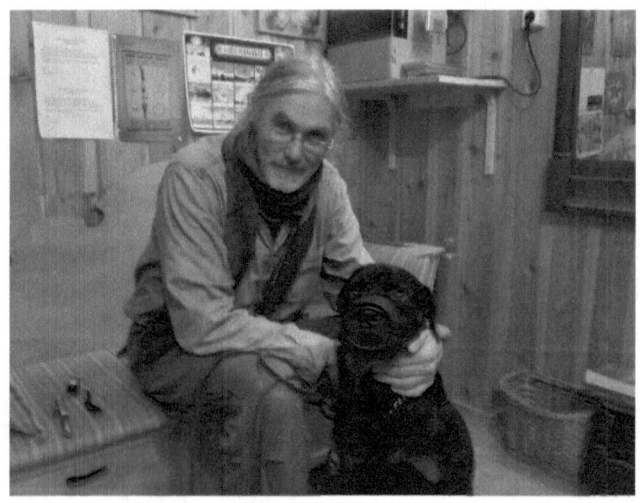

Hello,
send you as agreed a picture of you and Mighty.
I went and took blood tests today, these were compared with the first from 05.01.2014 and the result is positive and amazing.
I have a copy for you.
We look forward to coming to our appointment Wednesday 29.01.2014 kl.1430.

Regards Stein Unsgår

25. POSTSCRIPT

After the first printing of the Norwegian book "Har kreftens gåte en løsning" was published in 2014 followed by the English translation in 2016, I was informed by Are Thoresen that the treatment method, which is the main theme of the book had shown such an unexpected change in its effect. The TheMa Publishing Company descided to add an additional postscript to the 1ˢᵗ edition, in order to clarify the current situation.
The postscript is written by Are Thoresen.
FT

One major problem with the method, observed by Are Thoresen: The problem of "Translocation" of the cancer.

In most treatments of so called "Alternative medicine" the causes of the disease are usually just Translocated to other parts of the body, to other Organ-Systems or to other animals or humans.

This counts for acupuncture, zone-therapy, osteopathy, homeopathy and of course all of the treatments that have to do with massage, vitamins, minerals and food therapy.

 "Herrings law"[1] that is known within homeopathy and acupunctureis presented as a law of healing, which it is not. It is the

---

[1] *Herrings Law. This law states that cure occurs from; a). From above and downwards. b). From within outwards. c). Appearance of symptoms in reverse chronological order. This means: a); "From above downwards." Cure progresses from the head towards the lower trunk, that is to say the head symptoms clear first. With regard to the extremities, cure spreads from shoulder to fingers, or hip to toes. b); Cure starts from within outwards. Cure progresses from more important organs (e.g. liver, endocrine) to less important organs (e.g. joints). That is to say, the function of vital organs are restored before those less important to life. The end result of this externalization of disease is often the production of "treatment cutaneous rash". c); "Appearance of symptoms in reverse chronological order". More recent symptoms and pathology will clear before old, the disease "back tracks" so to speak. After the more recent problems have been cleared, it is not at all uncommon for the*

law of Translocation, which describes the Translocation within the body, but omits the Translocation to other entities within family, friends or animals.

How to avoid Translocation?

The first time I tried to treat the Middle, and only the Anatomical Middle, I was standing beside a horse together with **Dr. Markus Steiner**, a German college. Suddenly I *saw*, quite clearly with my Spiritual Eyes, the pathological structure in the stomach area of the horse, and another pathological structure in the area of the chest. With a violent shot from a "dermojet"[2] I then treated the exact middle between the two, and immediately they both pulled back. According to a college, **Dr. Markus Steiner,** the pathological structures did not entirely leave the body, but stayed in the front and the hind legs.

Since 2014 I have treated many human and veterinary patients following this method, using one needle carefully placed in the middle. Most of them are very satisfied with the great effect of this treatment. They describe strong energies changing and streaming through the body. Often these energies stream around in the shape of a lemniscate (the form of an "8"), and usually seek out the area of the body or the process containing the pathological structure and stream into this.

The patient feels this as a strong healing effect, and feels changed afterwards.

The Middle Point has really nothing to do with acupuncture, as I do not use any acupuncture point. I just put a needle between two areas of the body.

---

patient to experience the transient reoccurrence of old symptoms and pathology, which then disappears within a few weeks. Herrings Law, which is also termed the Law of Cure, is the logical inverse of the way in which chronic disease progresses both with regard to the patient himself and the ancestral history of the disease. The most important aspects of the Herrings Law are, "From within outwards" and "in reverse chronological order".

[2] **Dermojet** is a spring-loaded acupuncture "gun" that can shoot a liquid into the skin of most animals and men.

A description of the causes of cancer, the explosion of this disease today, why it is so difficult to heal and my (very) personal experiences in treating cancer.

All our diseases are caused by, or effectuated by the cooperation of different pathological structures inhabiting our bodies.
In cancer the cooperation of these structures is quite special, as they have joined closely together; there is almost no distance between them. This lack of distance between the structures makes it very difficult to heal as they have joined forces. It is much easier for them to stay put or if they have to translocate this is also quite problems for them.

In 1983 I realized that cancer had to be treated totally different from all other diseases. Most methods are more or less symptomatic, often just Translocating the pathology to other places or to other entities, humans or animals.

In 1984 I first applied "controlling" treatment method on a dachshund. The dog had mammary cancer (multiple tumors along the nipple line) and had begun to develop dyspnea (heavy breath) - it probably had several lung metastases. With acupuncture I treated the point labeled as LV03 (liver three), which strengthen the liver organ. In a few weeks the tumors had almost disappeared. The dog died several years later from a kidney deficiency.

In 1995 I treated for the first time a horse using the same method. The horse had been diagnosed with equine sarcoid, a kind of horse cancer. The result was very promising; the sarcoid disappeared within 6 weeks, and this was published in the journal of the Norwegian Veterinary Society, "Norsk Veterinærtidsskrift".

Since 1984, I have treated more than a 1000 patients suffering from all kinds of cancer, both animals and humans. The results have been especially good in mammary cancer (85%), also in melanosarcoma (80%). Results in lymphosarcoma and brain cancer have been moderately good (70%). However, my results in liver cancer and pancreatic cancer were mediocre; the healing rate being "only" 60% in the few patients I have treated.

As I started to try to avoid the translocation of the pathology, I tried to change the method to avoid this. In 2014 I then started to experiment with different methods, both the controlling method and the "Middle-point" method, especially within cancer treatment. Then something quite unexpected happened.

In cancer therapy the controlling treatment had worked very well for me for exactly 30 years.

The diminishing effect of the treatment method in 2014.

Then, in the period of spring 2014, it gradually ceased to work, or at least the effect lessened considerably. There was still an effect, the growth of the tumors decreased, but the real healing seen before was lost. Five of my closest students reported the same; the cancer-treatment-method gradually ceased working in the early part of 2014 even if both I and my students applied solely the well proven protocol (did not try to hinder the Translocation through applying the middle point). The method even ceased to work also for my students that were unaware of my experiments in trying to hinder the translocation. This did not happen to those of my students that had learned the method through reading my articles, only to those who had learned it directly from me. To find out if this change in effect also had affected my students, I posted the following neutral question on FaceBook in 2016;

"Have any of my students seen a change in the effect in the cancer treatment taught by me during the years 1984-2016".

A Belgian college wrote me this mail on the 3[de] of July after I had asked several colleges if they had noticed some change in the effect in cancer treatment during the last two years.

"Hello Are, as far as your question on cancer treatment is concerned my observations are the following: I do not remember if things changed two years ago, but I have noticed a general difference in reaction of patients.
Where the approach seemed to be simple, direct and effective

before, it seems as if it is different now. I can relate to a stomach cancer in a Labrador dog 10 years ago as an example. One needle once a month reduced the tumor from the size of a basketball to a Ping-Pong ball. It stayed in this state until the dog died two years later. Testing before each treatment revealed the same Meridian/organ complex involved and as a consequence the same acupuncture point was needled at each session. I noticed that it is not so anymore. Maybe it is to do with the location of tumors that makes a difference, or maybe it is me, but what I notice is that the tumor/cancer seems to try to "escape" the treatment protocol. For instance, last September I started to treat a cat with an osteosarcoma initiating in St01 (acupuncture point) right side. Testing before treatment involved Stomach Meridian/organ complex only. The owner is a colleague/friend and did not want to wait one month for the next session, so I saw the cat a week later for a check-up. This time the tumor seemed the same in shape and location, however .... it showed another Meridian involved when testing before treatment. I found a reaction in GB (Meridian) now and nothing in St (Meridian) anymore. The tumor tried to "escape" the Stomach Meridian and move to the GB01 (acupuncture point) position, so treatment needed an adaptation of strategy. During the last session last week, it shifted to SI (Meridian). I have seen this on several other occasions too for some time now, and even if the tumors stay under control, it seems to me that the reaction to treatment is not in the same straightforward way as it has been for all the previous years. I do not know what your observations are and why you send out the question, but I hope that my observations can be of some help to you.

Another college commented the following on the 2. of July 2016.

"The Middle-Point is the reason of any treatment done with Mistletoe, Viscum Album, Iscusin, Iscador, Viscum-Wala. Of course I have the tendency of recommending Wala medicaments. They were created by the orientation of Rudolf Steiner in order to increase immunological system - and in humans as all of us have an "I", the main point of any treatment is to strengthen Christ's forces. Often the point is not to live without the disease, nor is it to suffer

313

unbearably with the disease but to learn how to live with the disease and handle it. Anyway, Steiner was very clear that all researches on Viscum had to happen on a deep way as according to him, by using Viscum the need for surgery due to cancer would disappear. According to few medical doctor friends of mine, this will never happen. There is not enough money to run researches under anthroposophical guidance, and the allopathic Labs dominate the health research field in such a way that suffocates all forms of healing outside their approval. The more they control health decisions in all directions (WHO, State Controls of Medicaments and Diseases), the more distant is all possibilities to raise enough money to run good research with good results, accessible to all health communities and to the population in general. Unfortunately this is the hard reality. There is some research happening now but I have personal reasons to believe it will always represent loss and the institutionalized power is not open to loss.

Thank you, your feedback is just a marvelous fresh water stream. If you are 63 years old or more I dare to say your karma has been overcome and unless you create a new stream of treatment, your "I" will not anymore be the donator of healing forces or the carrier - as you also clearly see. It is necessary to create a new and even more innovative way to heal".

A college from Mexico wrote me this mail:

Dear Are. In the beginning, after you taught me the method, my results were great. Almost all cancers were healed. Then, about two years ago I started to experience mixed results, not always the best ones (remission).

This improved a little when I selected the acupoint by pulse resonance (according to Nogier) on the corresponding carpal or tarsal areas as you have described in your book. But after a while the results started to get worse again. I am curious about your personal experiences. I send you greetings from rainy Mexico City.

Notes

Introduction to the first edition:

Cf. http://www.hjernekraftverk.no/superstjerner, where the Norwegian Association of Researchers (NAR) has a promotion where they emphasize Norwegian research´s "superstars" - Norwegian scientists who have reached international acclaim. Moan is one of the first two researchers who have received this honor designation. In November 2013 he was presented in more than a full-page ad in "Morgenbladet".

[2] http://translate.google.no/translate?hl=no&sl=en&u=http://www.ous-research.no/moan/&prev=/search%3Fq%3Djohan%2Bmoan%2Bprofessor%2Bi %2Bmolekyl%25C3%25A6rbiologi%26biw%3D1093%26bih%3D558&sa=X&e i=RPS5UdaPCKGp4gS-xoF4&ved=0CEkQ7gEwBA

[3] The grossest example Moan mentioned, is that a summary of articles he has published internationally on vitamin D´s importance for prevention and treatment of cancer, was rejected by *the Journal of the Norwegian Medical Association*.

[4] Over twenty years later it is discovered and recognized that our immune system is much more fragmented and multifunctional than we have previously been aware of.

[5] Represents the highest level of publication of medical research

[6] In the qualitative test (one patient) in the hospital that the book documents, severe cancer development was stopped by two half an hour treatments before one managed to initiate hospital treatment - proven by biopsy, MRI, CT and PET CT images. The experiment was repeated twice, with equal sponaneous effect and documted in the same way.

[7] Many young cancer researchers today know parts of this knowledge and expect that it at some point will lead to radical changes in the understanding and treatment of cancer diseases.

[8] The Foundation Robin H. is managing this release and the next commercial release of the book, and is a guarantor that the project is a hundred percent ideal in the sense that profits from the sale is earmarked for new initiatives to spread awareness about the treatment method, including research- and treatment initiatives. The fact that the Foundation has been granted tax exemption for commercial activity, involves extra attention from supervisory- and tax authorities.

Foreword: (Not in the English edition)

[9] That the therapist has the same last name as the book's author, does not imply any familiar relationship, but is due to pure chance.

[10] Cf. Genreal information about RNA:
http://www.ntnu.no/doktorgrader/dr.philos/10.05/Snove.htm.

[11] The laboratory experiments can be studied here:
(http://www.sanare.no/studies.html) This link is deactivated by "someone" who probably not want the reaserch evidence to be linked).

Chapter 1:

[12] Pulse Diagnosis is a part of an ancient diagnostic method that still today are used by some acupuncturists to diagnose energetic imbalances in the body, deficiency or excess in organ processes or unsuccessful control of growth processes, often accompanied by strong growth processes, tumours or cancer.

Chapter 2:

[13] By this term I understand as the part of our health care system that holds both scientific authority and is authorized by our democratically elected supervisors. The so-called alternative therapists I see as a heterogeneous grouping which in reality represents the part of our health care system that does not have some form of authorization and in our society do not have any authority except what they can achieve in relation to the individual patients they treat. The term alternative implies an opposition or contrast as in many cases do not exist, if the individual therapist relate to health workers highest shared imperative, namely to help their patients to the best of their ability.

[14] The reason that I can not be more precise, is that the treatment method is communicated to an unknown number of therapists and clinics in the five continents. A few of them are referenced in the book's appendix.

[15] The Cancer Registry is the institution in Norway which disclose all relevant statistics - I thought until I discovered that the stats I was most interested in, an overview of trends in survival of the disease, is not published. I had to make it myself by putting together four other available statistics: average life of those who die of the disease, the number of diagnoses back in time corresponding average lifetime, the evolution of the number of diagnoses during this period and the number of deaths with cancer as the cause of death at the end of the period.

This work is described in Chapter 14 ("Statistics as a witness of truth"). The reason that the aforementioned statistics are missing, I do not know, but it is probably composed of different elements as illustrated in several of the chapters in this book's third and fourth parts. Because it is already revealed that the patient is still alive, this is one of the most exciting aspects I can offer. The second is naturally associated with which is introduced as a new, Norwegian and effective cancer treatment.

Chapter 3: [16] Thoresen emphasizes that what I basically refers to as "mutations" in connection with the precursor to cancer, is a popular description, and it's about

316

an *epigenetic* phenomenon: that genes can be active or inactive, turned on and off, depending on the environments influence. Since the level of precision here is adapted unskilled readers, it may be that I am using some widely understood, but professional imprecise concepts.

[17] There are of course many exceptions. I would especially like to highlight one of the most significant, Otto Heinrich Warburg (1883-1970, cancer researcher and Nobel laureate in medicine), who has presented compelling research on the causes of cancer. His research is only marginally been normative, which is currently rated by young researchers as highly regrettable. His fate may be due to that German disappeared as the leading scientific language after 1945, and that much German research was "forgotten" or underestimated by the World War II victors.

Chapter 4:

[18] An e-mail from Bruce Ferguson to Thoresen, which was sent him Dec. 6, 2013, is quoted in the appendix (Chapter 23: "Some examples of the method´s distribution") and is an example of how Thoresen´s treatment method is spread outside Norway.

Chapter 6:

[19] By own definition: One who search understanding primarily through thinking entirety as in that the parts reflect a larger whole, each part must not be thought of as separated or detached from the whole, and provides each part its specific mark, as opposed to an understanding that consists in partitioning (abstraction) and studies of the individual part separated from the other parts.

[20] It is also relevant to mention the acupuncture-meridians to be affected not only the points. The intention here is not to give any introduction to this treatment method´s technical details. Answers to the readers many "why´s?" must be sought from other sources.

[21] Quote from an article by Dr. Shen-Ying Zhang, a researcher at St. Giles Laboratory of Human Genetics of Infectious Diseases: *"White blood cells have long reigned as the heroes of the immune system. When an infection strikes, the cells, produced in bone marrow, race through the blood to fight off the pathogen. But new research is emerging that individual organs can also play a role in immune system defence, essentially being their own hero. In a study examining a rare and deadly brain infection, scientists at The Rockefeller University have found that the brain cells of healthy people likely produce their own immune system molecules, demonstrating an "intrinsic immunity" that is crucial for stopping an infection."* Cf. View the whole article: http://www.sciencedaily.com/releases/2012/12/121210221259.htm.

[22] That current cancer treatment has less healing power than most of us think, and that it is mainly limited to *prolonging life, but not to cure*, is documented in Chapter 14, "Statistics as a witness of truth".

[23] Which strategies that are effective in addition to the described acupuncture treatment, are described in Chapter 12: "Anecdotal healings and natural cancer treatment".

[24] In this case Manzetti has shown that novel peptides is formed in the blood of a breast cancer patient as a result of the acupuncture treatment Thoresen has developed for this patient-group. Manzettis further research with these newly discovered peptides, including on cancer cells *in vitro* (in glasstubes), and detection of the effective mechanisms of RNA- or mechanism attempts are reviewed in Chapter 11 ("Chi and chemistry. A meeting with the molecular biologist Sergio Manzetti").

Chapter 7:

[25] The conversation with Manzetti is placed in the book's third section "Chi and chemistry", where also the scientifical portion of Thoresen´s research is discussed in more detail.

Chapter 8:

[26] Duality should not be confused with dualism, cf previous note and below.

[27] Cf. *Veterinary Medicine: Complementary and Alternative Methods*, op.cit.:
"In Chinese Yin means the dark or non sunlit portion of a pile. Yang means the light or sunlit side of the mound or hill. The interaction between Yin and Yang is the most universal law/thought throughout the Orient. This law has its origin in a holistic world view, which thus relates to all conceivable phenomena. Just as modern quantum does, the Yin-Yang-law sees all phenomena containing two opposing forces, one that is necessary for the object at all to be able to consist.

This is not the same notion we can find in the older western dualism, where contradictions often want to destroy each other, and not to support or be a prerequisite for each other, and how they can exist without its opposite. Cf. Christianity, where good and evil are perceived as separate entities that can exist without each other.

In the East, contradictions are percieved as constantly changing, and tangled and prerequisite for each other. Yin and Yang are thus totally relative. Everything can be Yang in relation to something that is more Yin, so that all have something that is greater than themselves. Yin is more: under, the front, inside, cold, dark, feminine, night, hypo, descending, centripetal, diastolic passive. Yang is more: above, behind, on the outside, warm, light, male, day, hyper, rising, centrifugal, systolic, active.

The Yin-Yang symbol (cf. Last page of this chapter) is a good illustration of their relationships: The dark segment represents Yin, while the light represents Yang. These two segments waves or winds around each other dynamically and continuously transforms itself into its opposite. Within each segment represents the small dot that there is never any absolute: In all Yin there is some Yang and in all Yang there is some Yin."

[28] Cf. *Veterinary Medicine: Complementary and Alternative Methods*, op.cit.:

- *Jing Qi*: This energy comes from our parents and also from the whole cosmos in the moment of conception- and birth. It can also be "refreshed" throughout life through food and the like.
- *Inherited (Yuan-Qi)*: This form of energy is mostly deposited in the kidneys. It is responsible for a strong and long life.
- *Aquired (Zong-Qi from the air, Ying-Qi from the food)*: This form of energy is the life force that allows that we live and work. It flows through all processes and is supplied to us through food, water, air, smells, tastes.
- *Ehteric energy (equals Yuan-Qi)*: This is the energy that forms the basis for the structure of our organism.
- *Etheric body* is a term of the energy's structure. It is this structure that shapes our bodies, and that means we all have characteristics, that is, looks like we do.

Chapter 9:

[29] Source: NRK, samfunnsredaksjonen in the program "Sånn er livet" (such is life).

[30] Without knowing this with certainty, there is reason to assume that since these patients are severely debilitated, the drugs currently being tested, must be very strong and therefore have a significant risk of adverse side effects when applied to patients with normally functioning organs and yet not beeing severely immunocompromised.

[31] This term refers to numbers that are so inextricably linked to movable phenomenon, in this case, both the disease, the patients and less physical variables (varying) as *validity* and that precisely their absolute validity and significance is replaced by relativity.

[32] When I had familiarised myself a little deeper into the statistical material, I decided that the statistical probability that I would survive at the time of diagnosis, was closer to fifty to one than one to two. When considering the statistical probability that such a large tumour has metastasized. That it was not detected spreading at the time of the first images, may be due to the youngest cancer cells were the first to be defeated by the body's "cancer defense" after it had been stimulated by acupuncture treatment.

[33] After this was written, Wikipedia has entered a low incidence of "anecdotal healings", or as the mathematician would have termed random healings, as one of 100,000 cases of illness, ie 0.001%.

Chapter 11:

[34] Those who want to know more about Sergio´s genes and a little about him, can search the link http://en.wikipedia.org/wiki/Innocenzo_Manzetti#Family

[35] While the manuscript is prepared for publication, fall/winter 2013, it is initiated a scientific experiment with the method on 56 cancer dogs at Telemark University College.

[36] The modern scientific theory´s father, Karl Popper (1902-1994), put forward the idea of so-called negative verification of a hypothesis validity or correctness. According to him, a scientific theory is *not* finally proven, even if it is confirmed by observations by control experiments. Anytime it can be made an observation that does not fit in to otherwise well-established scientific "laws". Therefore, it is for Popper a methodological principle of all science that one should set the terms for how a theory of principle can be shown to be erroneous (ie how it can be falsified). A law or generalization (theory, hypothesis) that resists attempts at falsification, increase its acceptability or credibility. The more efficiently we are searching for falsification or possibilities for falsification, the more effectively we promote the growth of knowledge. In science it is in practice impossible to verify a public statement or a general law of nature in every possible cases where the statement could be applicable, it follows that science can never lead to a final truth or certainty, but only higher degrees of acceptability.

[37] The Radium Hospital´s initial review of the laboratory research are described in detail in Chapter 16: "An evaluation of Thoresen´s research".

[38] The most comprehensive study published on the effect of chemotherapy, was conducted in Sydney in 2004. It concludes that chemotherapy should be described as reliever of symptoms and neither is life-prolonging nor curative. The study shows that chemotherapy has only effect for 2.1 to 2.3% of patients in the United States and Australia which this study include within a 5-year period after treatment. If one had followed the patients over even longer, this percentage would have dropped further, possibly even down to no effect whatsoever with regard to the lasting survival from the disease (http://www.kreftbehandlinger.no/CellegiftStudien.pdf).

[39] Cf Thoresen's comments on the phenomenon of epigenetics: "It has been observed that the grandchildren of those who survived the Nazi concentration camps, utilize food better, and thus become easier obese. Similarly, changes in cancer genes after an acupuncture treatment are transferred to children and grandchildren. That way they will be better protected against cancer than their parents and grandparents. This effect is seen in dogs, where acupuncture treatment of females leads to smaller incidents of hip dysplasia for generations.
Epigenetics can also show and explain that the genetic characteristics can be modified for example by gender. One of the more investigated effects of epigenetics is found in Prader-Willis syndrome and Angelmans syndrome,

320

where the same piece of chromosome 15 may be missing in a child. If the missing piece comes from the father, ie with a spermcell, the result is Prader-Willi syndrome. Coming from the mother, the result is Angelman syndrome with different looks and symptoms compared with Prader-Willi syndrome. The mechanism and the explanation of this problem consists of an addition of a methyl group to a gene, which turns off the reading of the gene. Normal genes in maternal chromosome 15-bit is normally turned off, and if the corresponding bit is also missing with the father, the entire gene expression disappeares with respect to this piece of chromosome 15. This is also the case with Angelman syndrome, where it is the father's bit which is normally turned off. It can therefor play a role which parent the gene came from.

Such epigenetic changes may be due to connecting or disconnecting methyl groups or other regulatory elements such as acetyl groups or histones. Epigenetic effects have been observed in plants such as maize, in birds and mammals, and controls probably why connective tissue cells (fibroblasts) behave as fibroblasts and not as bone marrow cells, although the genetic material is the same. Effects from the mother seems more common than from the father. This may be why I find more similar acupuncture effects in mother and daughter than for father and daughter. And even less of the mother and son and the least similarity with father and son. "

[40] Source: Oslo Cancer Cluster from Aftenposten's special supplement on cancer in April 2010, regarding the price of developing cancer medicine.

Chapter 12:

[41] This happened decades before I was diagnosed with colon cancer. It is extensively described in the patient diary which content has been compiled and is sometimes quoted, and which I later hope to be able to adapt to a readable script.

[42] Unless these surprising and yet controversial conclusions seem sufficiently substantiated here, I show to that the scientific discovery that justifies Mæhlen statements, are a recurring theme in the book, and that cancer statistics through fifty years constitute the main argument that the discovery should be of crucial importance for future research and treatment.

[43] Nocebo means "I will harm". If we know that something can make us sick and we believe in it, we can actually get sick of it. This is called the noceboeffekten.

[44] One exception is preventive intake of vitamin D and to some extent, treatment with vitamin D. Several studies, the first from the United States and Canada in 2007, has shown that preventive treatment with vitamin D can lead to a reduction in cancer cases. This will be dealt with in more detail later in the chapter.

[45] Cf. http://translate.google.no/translate?hl=no&sl=en&u=http://www.ous-research.no/moan/&prev=/search%3Fq%3Djohan%2Bmoan%2Bprofessor%2Bi%2Bmolekyl%25C3%25A6rbiologi%26biw%3D1093%26bih%3D558&sa=X&ei=RPS5UdaPCKGp4gS-xoF4&ved=0CEkQ7gEwBA

[46] The studies are summarized by Paul Clayton in his book *Health Defence*, 2002 *How you can combine the most protective nutrients from the world´s healthiest diets to slow aging and achieving optimum health*

[47] For example, I met no other kind of approach to this complex problem than the question if I smoked, and how much alcohol I consumed.

[48] A proportion of the women had a cancer they were not aware of when they began the study. This is calculated statistically and deducted from the final result.

[49] Cf. http://www.aftenposten.no/nyheter/iriks/article1827469.ece.

[50] The article is based on the most extensive study conducted by the effects of chemotherapy, which was conducted in Australia and published in 2004. Cf. http://www.kreftbehandlinger.no/CellegiftStudien.pdf.
That in the United States, Australia and a number of countries on other continents are operateing with statistics showing survival after 5 years instead of one that shows the actual survival of the disease - when the very many cancer patients die much later than 5 years after diagnosis - will be thoroughly discussed in Chapter 14 ("Statistics as a witness of truth").

[51] Oslo, Universitetsforlaget, 1992.

[52] In a phone conversation Moan is describing this counter research´s insignificant both in quantity and in quality compared with the material he and his team have for inspection at the Norwegian Radium Hospital for those interested in vitamin D´s importance for our health.

[53] Cf. The description of the dogma of cancer as an irreversible disease earlier in this chapter.

[54] The reason that this notion is stuck in modern cancer researchers, is in my opinion due to that starting with the "discovery" of the cancer diseases solely focused on the disease´s final stages. There is little disagreement that once the disease has entered so far, it will without some form of intervention in such rare cases be improved or healed by self healing, that the term anecdotal healing and perception of the disease as irreversible here is accurate. That it is not until recently been conducted scientific research if this perception is correct or not, may be the reason why it has been today's young scientists that, based on the research in this field shows, that the disease's nature is dynamic.

Thoresen clinical results provide clear evidence that the effect of his treatment also applies to the disease´s last phases. It will in this case means that a large number of patients currently categorized as terminal, can be healthy if not tumours or side effects of hospital treatment has damaged vital organs or otherwise weakened the organism to such an extent that the patient dies even though the disease is retreating.

[55] Cf. note 35.

[56] Cf. http://www.budwigcenter.com/budwig-protocol.php regarding her diet and a Spanish center based on Budwig´s research. Since the description of the clinic in Stuttgart is not to be found on the Internet at the last review of the manuscript (January 2014), it may mean that it's closed down or possibly moved.

[57] Cf. http://www.nytimes.com/2006/01/10/science/10mirr.html?_r=1 for information about mirror neurons and the early beginnings of research on this phenomenon. You can also google *mirror neurons*.

[58] Cf. http://www.redjournal.org/article/S0360-3016(08)01216-9/fulltext and http://www.forskning.no/artikler/2008/september/196151.

[59]   Cf. http://www.pagepress.org/journals/index.php/ams/article/view/ams.2012.e11/pdf.

Chapter 13:

[60] An example of this is a program about sleep research that shortly before the time of writing, is shown in NRK´s "Schrødingers cat", and how sleep scientists were asked to examine the popular assertions (hypotheses) that coffee in the evening gave sleep problems, while moderate amounts of alcohol had the opposite effect. The researchers made an attempt at a sleep lab where they examined the sleep patterns of two people who took respectively alcohol and coffee shortly before the sleep phase. The results measured by electrodes attached to subjects, showed that both coffee and alcohol in different ways reduced sleep quality. In this case, it was not even conducted a cross-over trial in which subjects switched to who drank coffee, and who drank alcohol. The results were presented as fact, something not all researchers would necessarily have agreed upon, given that it was only performed one trial.

[61] By mapping the medication´s side effects it is taken into account if they are registered in as few as one in a thousand or more. Cf. The description of the effects in the PDR (*Felleskatalogen*: list of all medications that are allowed to be sold in Norway).

[62] There is a secondary, subordinate element of qualitative judgment upon approval of medications including regards to side effects. Similarly, it should in my view be an element of quantitative evaluation of a qualitative study before it is added a good enough transferability. Both are illustrated below.

[63] "The Study" in quotes because it is neither carried out by the hospitals that were responsible for the control, or scientifically submitted (published), but is a construction in retrospect based on the available facts from laboratory tests, MRI, CT, PET CT and the ongoing diary led observations of my own health. The summary is here briefly presented.

[64] Documented by patient-journal, oncologist Gustafson´s written report for the Norwegian Radium Hospital and also MRI, CT and PET CT late winter and spring 2008.

[65] Nevertheless, with my consent, but from the circumstances can not be understood otherwise than as being coerced.

[66] This is the oncologist assessment, quoted from the patient journal, and involves a stage of the disease that is regarded as absolutely incurable and where the hospital after this has only palliative treatment to offer patients.

Chapter 14:

[67] This applies to all major cancer forms. However, it achieved significant improvement in survival for some less common forms. It is particularly pleasing that this also applies to cancer in children.

[68] Source: NRK´s scientific editorial, Trondheim. A bit later, February 4, 2013, the Swedish Television program "Report" showed a report from the National Hospital in Stockholm, where a professor concluded that the withheld studies that are negative for drug manufacturers, in general, is the biggest problem related to the approval of pharmaceuticals in Sweden. I might add that American sites have pointed out that the cancer drug manufacturers can not reproduce the results of a majority of the studies that once ensured that the drugs were approved, and that, in other words, it is about a more systematic deception than those referred by NRK. This is a statement that can be true or false, and that I may have to leave to the special interested to verify. Nevertheless, it appears from the largest study conducted regarding the efficacy of chemotherapeutic drugs in Australia and the USA (and which I have previously referred to in Chapter 12 ["Anecdotal healings and natural cancer treatment"]) that the claims are correct. Anyway, this should be a field that those who accepts the use of medication in Norway, should take an interest in. We should have the assurance that our medications are approved through procedures that can not be suspected to be associated with serious offenses.

[69] Cf. http://wissen.spiegel.de/wissen/image/show.html?did=32362278&aref=image035/E0441/ROSP200404101600162.PDF&thumb=false.

[70] To ensure that nobody could doubt my numbers for survival, it's easy to test them. First, I found the latest available statistics for how many people have cancer as cause of death on the death certificate. In 2010, there were 11,036 people. As the incidence of cancer increases significantly every year, we must go back in time as many years as it takes on average from diagnosis to death for those who survive the disease, to determine the appropriate number of diagnosed that we can compare with. In 2010, there were 207,000 living with cancer, and with the average around 25 000 new diagnoses annually for the past 10 years we get closer to 9 years average survival for all cancers. We then compare the number of deaths in 2010 with the number of cancer diagnoses in 2002, which was 23 380 It provides 47.3% mortality.

[71] In 2008, the number of new breast cancer cases in Norway was 2 734. In the same year there were a total of 34,890 women suffering from breast cancer. To get a reliable picture of how long a breast cancer stricken woman living with this disease - whether she survives or dies from it - we must divide the total number of sick with the number of new cases in a year. The statistics for 2008 give us a good indication that the durations of the disease until this year was around 13 years *on average*. Since more women have the disease at a significantly shorter period, many must have the disease significantly longer than 13 years. A consequence of this is that statistics purporting to give an accurate picture of trends in survival of breast cancer, must extend over a significantly longer period than 13 years. Cf. the previously mentioned German survey covering 26 years.

[72] Cf. http://www.kreftregisteret.no/Global/Cancer%20in%20Norway/CIN_2010_with_Special_Issue_clustering_of_cancer_web.pdf.

[73] "Naive" is perhaps misleading here because it's about a belief in the future based on *erroneous* statistics that show progress. However, it is correct phraseology in comparison with the environmental disaster we may head towards. Also, I guess it is a kind of naivete to reason that including our previous Prime Minister, Jens Stoltenberg, is happy with what he *believes* is progress in the healthcare's effort to reduce cancer mortality.

Chapter 15:

[74] Here I associate the term coupling in the word's negative impact where there is disequilibrium in the "dividend", ie that the link is to benefit one party at the expense of the other. In this case - and in this chapter - takes the described connections, or mixing, consistent at the expense of ethics, and specifically at the expense of nation states (finance) and cancer patients (life and health).

[75] That it was until a new law in 2003 ("Law on alternative treatment" cf. http://lovdata.no/dokument/NL/lov/2003-06-27-64) was so, and that this partial withdrawal of the assumptions on the so-called quack law was based, allows us to categorize this as part of the "dark history" that modern medicine has behind itself, exemplified by bloodletting, electroshock, lobotomy and more. That the attitude has not changed appreciably since 2003, is the part of the dark prehistory which unfortunately highly are living among doctors and "most people" and is a great tragedy for those that it primarily affects, the so-called dying patients. For this group of patients the notion of cancer as irreversibility is a fateful dogma, which for the sake of just these patients should be removed through information campaigns and a shift of cancer care to a care that to a much greater extent than previously inspires cancer patients at all stages of the disease to lifestyle changes and possibly also seeking *natural cancer care including natural cancer treatment* as adjunctive therapy to the treatment the hospital at any time choose to offer patients.

[76] I want to emphasize what is said just above, namely that the hospital has not been able to help with the *disease itself*, which should be obvious, since surviving the disease are the patient's overriding purpose to seek treatment. This does not mean that hospitals have not helped patients in other ways, especially to improve the life expectancy. But in that one can never know if the general health degrading treatment are part of the factors that have been decisive for that the disease gets the upper hand, we face such an "obscured" problem complex that most of what is said and written, are fruitless speculations. This due to the fact that there are no research evaluating treatment in such a way that it is compared with an alternative or no treatment whatsoever. I am aware that this has ethical reasons. In the book, I have discovered ways to overcome these obstacles in the example in Chapter 12 ("Anecdotal healing and natural cancer treatment") and to refer to Hirnreise´s research on this patient group.

[77] "A large number" must be seen against the background that the hospitals themselves determine a terminal patient's chance of survival - by what they describe as anecdotal healing -, to 0 - zero - or 1 in a 100,000 cases (sources: oncologist Gustafson and Wikipedia). That Hirnreise interviewed about 600 patients who have survived a diagnosis of "terminal cancer patient", and then verify what they report as the cause of healing, confirms that the diagnosis is generally so inaccurate and not least so destructive that it should be replaced by information on the known strategies that can help the patient to get well even in this stage of the disease

[78] According to Ben Gold Acre in the book *Bad Science*, 2012 - a media known critic of all that purports to be science - the largest American pharmaceutical manufacturers has a profit of 1 200 billion crowns per year.

[79] The following link shows examples of stealth marketing hat is revealed: http://dgesel.wordpress.com/2009/08/10/hello-world/. However, there remains the question of which methods have not yet been revealed.

[80] 4th of February 2013 SVT Rapport showed a report from the National Hospital in Stockholm, where a professor concluded that the withheld studies that are negative for drug manufacturers in general, is the biggest problem related to the approval of pharmaceuticals in Sweden. I might add that American sites have focused on that the cancer drug manufacturers can not reproduce a majority of the studies that once ensured that the drugs were approved. In other words, it's about a more systematic deception than those previously reported by NRK. This is especially regarding a relatively new flood of drugs with the popular term "happy pills" or antidepressants. In this case it has been revealed that the least favorable studies conducted before the approval of the drugs were kept secret. A consequence of this is that new studies after a few decades of use shows that the medication has no demonstrable beneficial effect on more than one in five patients. It may also be appropriate to recall the largest study conducted on the effect of chemotherapeutic drugs in Australia and the United States (cited in note 64), and where it is found only lasting effect of no more than 2% of cancer patients given these drugs.

[81] It is in Germany, the fight against the directive has been strongest, and where it is carried out such calculations. The reason is that alternative and natural medicines have a very different distribution here than in most other EU countries. Because of the directive a significant share of cancer patients to be referred to the black market in order to continue with their medication, that they - rightly or wrongly - is convinced will help them in the fight against disease and death. This assumes that the directive really is being followed up by the players on this market and the authorities to enforce it. Given the EEA agreement, the directive also applies in Norway.

[82] In contract research can economically ties to a client easily cause the researcher choosing other priorities than he had done if he had been working for a public or institutional client.

[83] Phase two of the clinical trial usually occurs with about 200 people. If this shows a significant effect, the trial is terminated with larger randomized trials to better identify the drug's side effects.

[84] For obvious reasons it has been impossible for me to verify the exact number of these studies and their quality. For a summary I refer to Paul Clayton's book *Health Defence*. Cf. note 46.

[85] NRK P2, "Sånn er livet", october 2010 (now "Ekko").

Chapter 16:

[86] The reason this has not yet been able to happen extensively in his home country, it is given a few examples in this chapter, but especially in the book's epilogue, where I compare the events that took place six months before the book's printing with a form of hidden warfare. Readers may themselves judge from the documentary resume, but it is not difficult to realize the purpose of the war.

[87] Here and some other places in the chapter it is referenced events far back in time. This has meant that I have had to make some choices with regard to chronology.

[88] So-called peer review. Cf. "Cancer and the Hidden Tradition: Is There a Role for Acupuncture Beyond Adjunctive", *Medical Acupuncture* (number 1, 2011). This article is cited in this book's appendix.

[89] The article should in my view arouse interest among professionals with respect to scientific publications in the highest graded journals. They namely never publish articles that are not thoroughly verified, in terms of both the content and the author, and are not considered innovations within the relevant field of research.

[90] In the recent review of the manuscript I remembered that I only had the dog owner's word that squamous cell carcinoma is incurable, and therefore seached online. In addition to descriptions of the disease I also came over a for me unknown

website: http://www.madamim.net/_Old_MadaMim/ArtikkelFanta-HTML/ArtkkelFantaMai2007.html!

[91] When the word study is used in the text, it is with expressed reservation that it must be regarded as amateurish. Thoresen also disclaim liability for use of the title "scientist" about himself. This can have several meanings. Not least, it implies a formal qualification he does not have.

Chapter 17:

[92] Cf. Møller´s Doctorate, which describes the increase in the number of cancer cases. (Cf. Chapter 14: "Statistics as a witness of truth".)

[93] Most known from animal feed, but also from the tobacco industry, where smokers are more dependent on substances other than nicotine to such an extent that it helps them little to be offered other brands than just what they are addicted to, if the stores are out of "their" brand. Then they rather walk a mil to the nearest tobacco outlet.

[94] These statistics are described in detail in Chapter 14 ("Statistics as a witness of truth"). What follows in this section is a simplified impact analysis based on the new picture that form from modern cancer treatment´s effectiveness after it was realized that the "old image" is a forgery based on 50 years of systematic misinformation.

[95] It will probably also dampen the discussion that acupuncture has no effect when it can be detected in the blood sample that *something* happens, and that this *something* can be proven in the laboratory to have an effect on bacteria, viruses and other micro-organisms that have caused health problems.

[96] "Only" in this context is a relative term. It shows that the breakthrough prior to the publishing is done, but the discovery will also require much additional research, including by other researchers. This is not "peanuts" getting approval for in the current situation. I hope and believe the discovery could pave the way for future research in publicly controlled and paid research if - or hopefully when - the method's effect on cancer to a greater extent is being recognized.

[97] See an explanation of this a few pages further on in the text and note 88.

[98] That is, in cases where the removal of the tumour by surgery is not considered to have a healing effect because the tumour for example, too much has infiltrated surrounding organs or other tissues (the category I was in before Thoresen for the third time stopped the cancer development and made the tumour to shrink, so that at the next CT and MRI it was no longer problematic to remove it).

[99] It should be noted that not all patients respond to acupuncture treatment, which according to Thoresen is a general uncertainty with all acupuncture treatment.

[100] Cf. For example, the PhD Candidate Jill Hervik at Vestfold Hospital, taking her doctorate on the subject of "acupuncture treatment in hospitals". During a meeting in October 2012, she oriented me about a research project that has resulted in that the hospital for several years has used an acupuncture treatment that involves more than just relieving pain. The treatment is based on similar processes as those underlying Thoresen´s treatment, by stimulating the body's capacity for self-healing. Hervik could tell that there are two reasons for such a radical step onto the bridge between Eastern and Western medicine, which constitutes a review of the topics in this book:

- A study conducted at Henry Ford Hospital in Detroit and presented at the European Breast Cancer Conference in Berlin, April 2008,
- and a smaller study conducted at Vestfold Hospital by Jill Hervik and Odd Mjåland, surgeon at the South Coast Hospital, Kristiansand

Cf. note 55 and 56.

[101] Cf. chapter 4: "Who is Are Thoresen?"

Chapter 18:

[103] Cf. http://www.etablererkontoret.no/manedens-etablerer/margit-buen-bor-pa-en-liten-gard-i-ovre-bo-hvor-hun-na-er-i-gang-med-a-utvikle-sin-egen-virksomhet-hun-har-hatt-eget-firma-i-noen-ar-som-hun-har-drevet-ved-siden-av-utdanningen-men-na-onsker-h-2/, and www.margitbuen.no.

[104] With a little good will and extra round numbers can the misleading statistic the Cancer Registry publishes called "Survival" be interpreted as Stoltenberg does. The problem is not a generous rounding, but that the Cancer Registry´s statistics as shown in Chapter 14 ("Statistics as a witness of truth") does not show anything about how many people survive cancer, but just how many who survive at least five years after diagnosis. The average remaining life *of those who die of the disease, is nearly nine years*. So still only 1 of 2 survives cancer or more accurately 52.3% (by my calculations).

[105] Thoresen has no other influence on the study than that he performs the actual treatment of the dogs. The experiment is led, monitored and evaluated by independent experts, whose task is to recognize the scientific qualifications so that it can be the subject of an objective scientific study.

[106] Cf. www.hjernekraftverk.no

[107] According to Skavland, a permanent guest in NRK when unauthorized medicine is to be discussed, 76% of Norwegian cancer patients survive the disease, which is just over 3 out of 4. And not 2 out of 3, as our previous Prime Minister claimed in his campaign, or 1 out of 2, which is the bare fact.

Where does Skavland have his numbers from? I challenge him to elaborate, to NRK and all of us who trusts both the radio and the annual general practitioners. That I choose such a method, is not alone due to his misinformation, but that he is a grateful example of professionals who themselves do what they accuse colleagues whose opinions differ from their own to do, namely to present figures and claims they do not have scientific covering for.

Although Skavland expressly said "in Norway", I suspect him to refer the American statistics, as of recent years meant that the United States suddenly did apparently much better than all European countries with regard to the results of cancer treatment. This is due to an even bolder manipulation with cancer statistics than the Norwegian Cancer Registry has been doing. Both are described in detail in Chapter 13, "Statistics as a witness of truth".

Chapter 19:

[108] The key experiment descriptions from Ann Arbor are unfortunately not longer available online, but can be obtained from Are Thoresen – arethore@online.no..

www.ingramcontent.com/pod-product-compliance
Lightning Source LLC
Chambersburg PA
CBHW021419170526
45164CB00001B/21